Scripture quotations marked (NLT) are taken from the Holy Bible, New Living
Translation. Copyright 1996, 2004, 2015 by Tyndale House Foundation. Used
by permission of Tyndale House Publishers, Inc., Carol Stream, Illinois 60188.
All rights reserved.

Printed In the United Stares of America

TABLE OF CONTENTS

Introduction 1

Most Important Chapter 3

One Meal A Day (OMAD) 23

Things You Can Have Fasting With OMAD: 29

What is a "Tasting?" 30

Two Tastings and a Meal 32

The Eating Window 39

What is Keto Flex? 45

Better ROI 47

Is it Worth It? 49

How Am I Going to Feel When I Eat This? 50

Hunger and Fullness 51

Identify True Hunger 52

SKIP, SWAP, or BITES 55

Wait for Your Stomach to be Empty 58

Use the Three-Bite Rule 60

Hara Hachi Bu 65

Savor Your Food 67

Ways to Avoid Overeating 69

Mindset 74

How to Get a Mindset Reset: 79

Extended Fasting 85

INTRODUCTION

I am so grateful for all of the friends who I have interviewed and who have put up with me asking the same questions over and over.

I would like to thank Missy Owens, Kim Hinton, Andrea DiGeronimo, Laurie Baggett and so many other thin women who have really helped me understand at, a deeper level, what a thin eater eats. With their guidance, I feel like I keep learning more and more about the thoughts and mindset of a thin eater. I have so many people who have been so gracious and opened up to me and I am grateful to all of you!

My top priorities in life are to be a great mom, a great wife, a great businesswoman, and a great friend. I want you to know that I am not perfect, but I am in such a better place than I was years ago. When it comes to learning how to eat, you often have to take four steps forward and three steps back and keep going until you get to that place where you are happy. In the past, I would hear about the latest diet that everyone was trying, and I would say to myself, "I just can't do it." I know what it's like to have food as your best friend and as a comfort. I have been there and done that again and again. I understand feeling hopeless. I know what it's like to starve myself and then overeat. I would constantly try a new diet, and my day would be made or ruined by what I ate. I used to deprive myself and would go into this cycle: deprive, crave, binge. All that changed when I decided that no food was off-limits, and I replaced it with thoughts of eating the most delicious, clean foods, without being overly obsessive.

All of these women that I have interviewed had the following in common:
- ✔ Do not count calories.
- ✔ Do not count carbs in detail.
- ✔ Do not obsess over everything they put in their mouth.
- ✔ Do not Yo-Yo diet.
- ✔ Do not have meal plans.
- ✔ Do not measure every little bit of food that goes in their mouth.

As a result of my time with them, I can now say that I do not binge on food anymore and I rarely overeat. The goal of this book is to help other people break free from being tormented by food. I am not a nutritionist, I'm a woman who has been where you are and took some time to question those who were where I wanted to be. I am however an expert on intermittent fasting because of the years I have spent researching, interviewing thin women, and applying the principles that I learned to obtain my goals.

Waist Away was the beginning of the story, and this book is the continuation. When I wrote that book, I had only been living some of the principles for a few short months. All of the principles are still applicable, although, in this book, I dive much deeper! I now realize that I didn't totally understand some of the concepts when I wrote that first book. For instance, I now understand that eating two full-sized meals per day was actually more food than I really need. The more you use these tools, the more they become second nature. You can be the girl who can just eat three French fries and not eat anymore (trust me, I do it!). If you haven't already read *Waist Away the Chantel Ray Way*, I hope you will give it a read. If you've already read it and are continuing with this one, you will learn to eat like a woman who is intuitively thin without even thinking about it.

There are some things I am still not good at, but I watch my thin friends and I get better every single day. I encourage you to read this book over and over until the ideas become second nature to you. If you haven't read *Waist Away the Chantel Ray Way,* I encourage you to do so. You can also listen to my podcast at https://chantelrayway.com/chantelrayway-podcast/ or visit https://chantelrayway.com/ for tons of free resources to assist you on this journey.

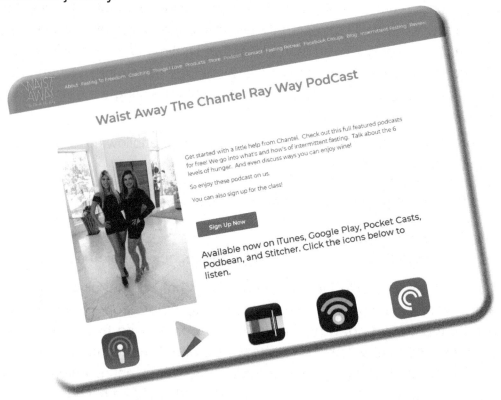

Most Important Chapter

This chapter is the most important chapter of this *entire* book! I'm going to give you a brief overview of what you can expect to be discussed in detail as you read this book. Even though I'm giving you this overview, it's absolutely crucial that you read the entire thing, because a lot of times what happens is you read a portion and then you go "OK, I get the gist of it!" and then you stop reading. This is where I went wrong with my interviews. When I interviewed people, I learned 80% of it and wrote it in my first book. I realized that I missed valuable information after I had already written it.

I almost entitled this book *Intuitively Thin Habits* because one of the things people who are successful do is consistently demonstrate the disciplines that other people only show occasionally. Let me give you an example: some people save a little bit of money and then they start going crazy buying large items and big cars that they can't afford. However, people who are financially wealthy make sure that they are continually making wise investments and *sometimes* they splurge. Overall, they are consistently making the wiser choice. I believe that one of the habits that thin people do intuitively; they look at their eating on a weekly basis instead of daily. For example, if they have a bad day and eat more than they wanted to, they just make it up the next day or later in the week.

Everyone always says, "I need a specific meal plan to follow to stay thin." Remember, there is *no* meal plan. One person may feel horrible after they eat avocados, but avocados are healthy and lots of thin people eat them all the time. In my last book and probably somewhere in my podcast, I may have said something like, "I don't eat a lot of grains or beans." I get the question a lot asking, "what is wrong with grains and beans?" There are a lot of thin people who eat grains and beans and still do intermittent fasting. I do occasionally eat them, but I don't feel my best when I do. I do more of a Keto-flex diet where I add a sprinkling of grains and beans into my diet sporadically. I tend to focus on eating with fruits, vegetables, and items with lots of protein. That is just how I feel my best, so you have to customize what you eat to feel your best.

This is what thin eaters do all the time! They are consistently doing things that heavier people only do occasionally. They make small decisions that make a big difference over time. That is what that my friend Kim says is her number one thing to do: be consistent over time.

Habits matter and one of the things that you'll learn are the habits of these intuitively thin eaters. We realize that what we do to our body will be a reflection on what we will do continually, not just for a couple of days.

I remember reading a statistic somewhere on Google that said over 90% of the New Year's resolutions that people make aren't in effect by the end of January. **90%!** That means only 10% of people actually follow through! That is just crazy!

One of my biggest concerns is that you're going to read a section and hear that sometimes I eat half of a donut, and then you'll take that and go, "OK I can do that too." Part of being thin is not eating half a donut every day! One of the things you will learn in this book is that thin eaters eat in a keto flex diet. They sprinkle their diet with decadent food choices. The keyword is *sprinkle*!

The other thing that people do is focus on the WHAT, but they don't focus on the HOW they got there. They also focus on WHO they want to be. So, for me, I had to look at myself and say, "I want to be an intuitively thin eater, I want to consistently consider what a thin eater does," and that's what motivated me to keep asking them over and over what they do.

If you think about it, every person wants to be physically fit. I've never met anyone that was like, "You know what, I just really want to be three or four hundred pounds." Being physically fit is everyone's goal. If we all have the same goal, then why do some people achieve it and some people don't? Every one of the NFL football teams says, "We are going to win the championship this year!" But some achieve it, and some don't. We have to look at why you will or will not be able to achieve your goal. The answer lies in inconsistency.

I see people all the time that are like, "Wow I gained 50 pounds! I don't know how that happened" or "I gained 20 pounds and I didn't even notice, it just crept up on me!" Here's what I see heavier people do all the time: they will eat salad and other healthy meals for three days in a row, and after the three days, the scale doesn't move. You hear them say, "I'm just going to eat whatever I want, this isn't working" and they give up. As you know, I didn't lose any weight for over three weeks when I first started doing intermittent fasting! The third week I lost 6 lbs! I have seen people who do intermittent fasting for two days, maybe they had a lot of salt, and they get on the scale and they gained two pounds and they go, "this doesn't work" and then they quit.

When you don't see the results you want, avoid going into an attitude of saying, "Oh forget it, I'm going to go eat half of a cake!" Or maybe you eat a third of the cake all in one session and you don't gain any weight, so then you incorrectly conclude that bad decision didn't really move the needle that much. When you don't see results fast enough, you mistakenly conclude that small, good decisions don't matter that much. This is a *big* mistake! A small change or a small tweak that you do every day does make a big difference. When you quit, you miss out on the truth that our lives are the culmination of all those small decisions, and that all those small little decisions matters. That's the piece I really missed the first time around that I want to teach you this time.

One of the things the thin eaters say is that they eat in the same patterns every day and every week! For instance, making the small decision that you are going to have black coffee instead of coffee with tons of cream and sugar!

The Bible says, "do not be weary by doing good but at the proper time we will reap a harvest." I just started gardening, (which I hate by the way). I never realized how long these little seeds take to grow a little mini cucumber. It takes a while to reap that harvest! You can't be impatient.

The best way for you to be consistent is for you to have accountability. To help you with this, we have private coaching and group coaching at https://chantelrayway.com/coaching or you can join our Facebook accountability group!

You will see that a lot of the things I am going to share I follow on a daily basis. One of the things I really struggle with is eating slowly. To fight this, I have to remind myself about the Parasympathetic Nervous System. Our nervous system has two primary parts that are crucial to understanding. First, one of the things that my podcast guests have told me (in addition to slowing down when I'm eating) is to reduce my stress when I am eating. Thin eaters predominantly eat at night when things are calmer. So, when thinking about what time is best for your eating window, you should decide on a time you are not too stressed to eat. For me, when I am at work, I am stressed most days. Another thing my podcast guests have told me is that the Sympathetic Nervous System controls our "fight or flight" response, and the Parasympathetic Nervous System controls our "rest and digest" response. We always want to eat when we are in a parasympathetic state.

Our sympathetic nervous system kicks in whenever we are experiencing any kind of real or perceived threat. If fear, real or imagined, shows up in your thoughts or environment, (ie, being chased by a fox in the woods, running late for a plane, or trying to finish a never-ending to-do list at work) our sympathetic nervous system kicks in. Think about this: Digestion is not essential when we are fighting for our lives. If we find ourselves in massive stress response – like if a lion was chasing us – **our digestion completely shuts down**. In our world, that lion chasing us might be "having a strict deadline for work and being completely stressed out." It would make total sense, if we *did* have a lion chasing us, why would we need massive digestive enzymes to be kicking in at that time? Even judging ourselves for eating four cookies in one sitting — we activate our Fight/Flight response and shift into a stress zone.

Remember:

We don't want to get goals that are "do goals," we want "who goals"!

WHO DO I WANT TO BE IN MY WEIGHT LOSS?

For me, I want to eat like an intuitively thin eater that never goes on a diet *ever* in her life! I want to break free of diet jail! I never want to have foods to buy, I never want to count calories or count points! I want to control my portions and satisfy my hunger! I only want to eat when I'm physically hungry and I want to recognize when I am truly hungry, instead of eating for emotional reasons! I want to obey God and I never want to overeat!

You have to put systems in place to be successful and in this book you're going to hear systems that some of the thin women use that make them successful. The number one system they use is eating one meal and a tasting, every once in a while one meal, and sometimes one meal and two tastings. The majority of what they eat is a keto flex diet, without knowing that they are eating that way, and sprinkling their meal with some decadent foods they love.

Remember:

What your end goal is. Who do you want to be?

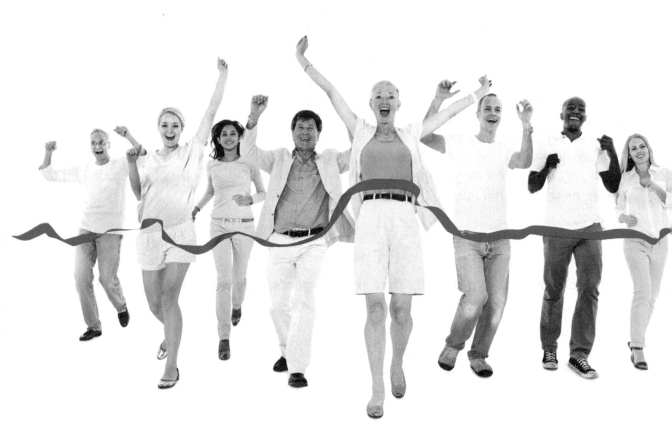

If so, you have to fix your daily habits.

Download my podcast "Waist Away Through Intermittent Fasting" and listen to the podcast on habits for more in-depth tips.

I want to share with you some conversations I have had with some of my friends. We will dive deeper later in the book, but this will give you some insight into the lives of women that I respect and value, who happen to be thin eaters! I believe that people learn from real stories and from real people. These people are as real as it gets!

My friend Andrea is one of the few thin people I know who have a longer eating window. At 9 a.m. she is eating her tasting in the morning and then she eats dinner at night. She usually skips lunch. Because of this, she will sometimes do two tastings. She will do something really small in the morning, like a quarter of a banana, four strawberries, and three nuts. That's how little she is eating in the morning. In the summer, she only does one meal and a tasting because she wants to be thinner in the summer for bathing suit season!

For me, one of the things that I did to lose a lot of weight is intermittent fasting by eating in a six-hour window. I still have more weight that I want to lose, but it's because I was eating two meals a day that I failed to lose the weight. The only way for me to get to the weight I want is to do one meal and maybe a tasting, depending on how big that one meal is. Where I went wrong was eating two meals in that six-hour window. And the other thing is, if I ate too much at lunch, I should not have a tasting at dinner, I wasn't physically hungry. That's the difference these women did: if they have too much at lunch, they don't have a dinner! That's a big deal. This is going to be mind-blowing to you! Go to Google and search for weight and calories. You will see that it's like 40 calories or more per five pounds. Again, I am not counting calories, but some charts show you the calories needed to lose five pounds is a very small amount of food. It can be the difference in eating an extra half of an apple a day that can make you five pounds heavier. And again, I AM A BIG PROPONENT of not counting calories. But sometimes I must mention this to open up people's eyes. The smallest amount of extra food could be keeping you from being the weight you want to be. Thin eaters are cognizant of calories. They know that avocado is high in fat and calories, but it is also so great for you. They will not eat two whole avocados in a sitting! I can tell you I have probably eaten more than two avocados while eating guacamole, but again I have to be mindful to not eat too much and let it get out of control.

What is important to note is that none of these women are counting calories. I have provided the approximate calorie count for context, but I assure you they aren't counting calories. When asked what this looks like on a day-to-day basis, my friend Missy said, "At 1 p.m. I wanted chicken tenders, so I had one and a half chicken tenders over top of a salad. Another day for my tasting I ate one piece of toast with an egg and a slice of bacon. But, both nights at dinner, I had protein and non-starchy vegetables. It's probably about 300 calories for my tasting. One night I might eat onions, mushrooms and eat half of steak. Another tasting I would make pickled vegetables and arugula salad with hummus. It's either a salad with a protein or half of a sandwich or an open-faced sandwich. I only eat one slice of bread with whole grains. Then at dinner, I will have protein and veggies. I eat what I want, but I eat a lot of veggies." Over and over the stories are consistent, "I eat one meal at night, and I eat something 200-450 calories for my lunch." Even though they never know how many calories it is. One of the reasons they almost all have lunch as a tasting and dinner as the meal is because they want to have a lot of energy during the day. Digesting food takes a lot of energy. They have enough during lunch, so they don't go crazy at dinner.

So, if you look at how many calories these women are eating it's approximately 1,400 to 1,500 calories a day. They're having about, you know, 1200 calories in their dinner and about 300 calories in their tasting. It isn't that thin women actually pay attention to *counting* their calories, but they are aware of when they are actually hungry, eat what they want, have a small tasting instead of a midday meal, and don't overeat.

I would ask someone, "What do you eat and what time do you eat?" Nine times out of ten they would say, "You know, I'm just not a big breakfast person. I never eat breakfast, so I start eating around 1 o'clock and then I usually eat dinner around 5:30 p.m. I pretty much finish around 6:00 p.m." I would ask another person and she would say, "I start eating a snack around 2:00 p.m., I'll have something small, and then I will have dinner around 6:30 p.m." After interviewing them more in-depth, I realized that all of them were eating one medium-size meal and a snack or "tasting". For example, when I asked my friend, Laura, "What did you eat yesterday?" she remarked that she had a big lunch and said, "You know I was full, so I didn't eat anything the rest of the day!" This is a perfect example of how I would have watched her eat that big meal, and in my mind, before I would say, "See she can eat whatever she wants and still stay so thin!" But I didn't realize that's all she ate for the whole day. I would eat exactly what she ate but then go home and eat dinner and be like "Why am I not thin? I ate exactly what she did!" When in reality, I had eaten so much more.

As I began to dig deeper, I realized what all of these thin women were doing: not only are they doing intermittent fasting, but it seems like they were just having one meal and a tasting or just one meal some days! I realized that the thinnest girls naturally eat this way.

The other piece is asking the question: "What are you deciding to eat?" One of the biggest questions they ask themselves is: "How am I going to feel about myself after I eat this?" The second is: "How am I going to feel physically after I eat it - Is this worth it?" Almost every person I would interview would say, "If I have a carb or bread for lunch, I would not be having rice or potato for dinner." Not because they don't want another serving of carbs, but rather the excess carbohydrates would make them feel overly full. They might have one slice of bread on an open-faced sandwich for lunch, and salmon and veggies for dinner. They might have a burger with no bun and then eat some fries and shrimp and vegetables for dinner. For lunch, they might have a grilled chicken salad and then dinner is maybe rice and chicken and broccoli. I'm beginning to see a trend here! They all say, "I don't like to be too full after I eat!" 100% of the woman I interviewed always said they don't like to be too full because they feel tired and have no energy if they eat too much.

"This, That, or Bites of Both." I am going to talk about that several times in this book. This is how thin eaters eat. Thin eaters are not getting pasta, bread, and dessert! They are either getting pasta, or bread, or dessert. If by chance they want to get all of them at one meal, then they only have 3 bites of pasta, 3 bites of bread, and 3 bites of dessert! But they normally don't do this. It is this, that, or bites of both.

I tried to make it catchy so you can say it every time you are making a decision. Should I have this or that? Or do I want bites of both?

When I asked one of the thin eaters why she wouldn't have alcohol and dessert together, she would say that would be like eating a double whopper at Burger King. They don't do the double Whopper, they don't do alcohol with sugary desserts, they don't do a high carb pasta and a sugary dessert. They choose either this or that, or fun size bites if you want to get into the fat burning zone.

This is especially true when it comes to sugar, carbs, and alcohol. I asked all of the thin women that I interviewed about how much sugar they eat. They said, "I might have 50 cals of something sweet -like two chocolate candy kisses after I finish my meal." Or others would say instead of doing something little each day, they might have one dessert at the end of the week on a Saturday night. Some of the very thin women might say, "I might have a dessert every other week if I really really want it! One of the thin girls said, "If I do eat a dessert, I don't also have alcohol within a 24-hour span... I look at things in about a 3-to-7-day window of time as far as how much sugar, carbs and alcohol I have been eating."

This was an aha moment for me. None of the girls would really eat dessert every day. Some of them might've had two bites every day of something sweet, while another one had nothing during the week, but then on Saturday they might have 3/4 of a dessert at a nice restaurant, and the real skinny ones might've had half a dessert every other week.

If you are eating too much sugar, the sugar is going to interfere and stop you from getting into that fat burning zone.

When I asked the thin eaters about maintaining their lifestyle, every single person that I interviewed would say the same thing: "You know if I gain three or five pounds more than I would like, I just stop eating sweets and have a little less carbs for a week or two, and that will help me lose the weight that I want. Then I can introduce sugar and carbs back in small amounts."

One thing that I have found will really hinder me from losing weight is having too much vegetable juice and fruit juices. I really try not have fruit juices, except for maybe a splash of cranberry juice in my water. For me, juice really spikes my insulin and I have to be really careful with it. The one juice that I have to drink because my electrolytes can get off is coconut water. Even with coconut water, I try to only have about a half of a cup. Everyone in my office knows that if I am really not feeling great, a half a cup of coconut water makes me feel like a new person. There is only one brand I like, Nirvana brand, and it's made from real young living coconuts. Otherwise, I can only drink it straight out of an actual living coconut.

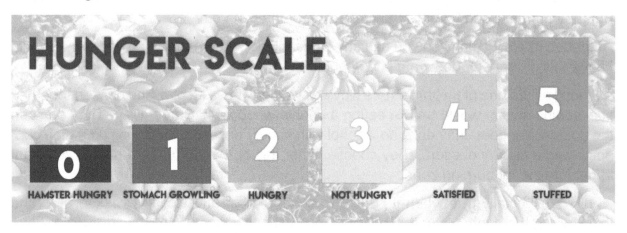

HUNGER SCALE

0	1	2	3	4	5
HAMSTER HUNGRY	STOMACH GROWLING	HUNGRY	NOT HUNGRY	SATISFIED	STUFFED

The other aha moment that I really had was just how few times a thin eater is eating sugar. What I realized is they are having about 50 calories of sugar per day, meaning half of a cookie, two small Hershey kisses or they're having 3/4 of one big dessert maybe once a week or maybe every other week. Sugary desserts throw out so much of your fat-burning, that it's really really important that you limit it as much as possible. Now when we look at the hunger scale, if you think about it, most people eat dessert when they are at a level four on the hunger scale. But people who are thin, save room for dessert. They might eat until they are at a 3.7 on the hunger scale and then maybe a desert every now and then to take them to a max of 4.0 on the hunger scale. Again, they only do this every now and then and this was what I got wrong in my first book. What I have found is that most over-eaters wait until they're a 4.2, and then say, "I'm going to have something sweet that puts me to a 4.6."

In my first book, I said that you could have something decadent maybe three bites of it once or twice a day, but honestly that is just too much! As I'm interviewing more thin people, they aren't having that kind of sugar every day, they are really limiting how much sugar that they can have.

I'm going to make a chart so you can see how much sugar is in some of these foods and how this is going to stop you from getting into fat burning if you were overdoing it.

The other thing that thin people do is they will often have fruit if they want something sweet and that will kind of curb some of their sugar desire. Let's look at some examples of what you can eat instead some of your favorite sugary desserts.

Let's look at a Snicker's bar. With the amount of sugar and calories in one candy bar, you could eat approximately 3.5 peaches.

One slice of chocolate mousse pie is about 300 calories which is the same as eating 3 apples or 4.2 slices of Dave's Killer Thin Sliced Bread.

One Snickers bar's calories has the same amount of calories as 8 cups of raw broccoli.

One slice of cheesecake has the same amount of calories as 80 almonds.

The way that thin people eat their chocolate is they literally take a tiny piece and savor it. I was watching my friend Christie eat a piece of chocolate, and she will take a piece and let it melt into her mouth, giving the chocolate a minute to melt and savor that piece. Then, she will put in another piece, and in the end, she's eating just a few pieces of dark chocolate. My mother likes to eat these organic chocolate chips, she will take a small handful put them in her hand eat a few chocolate chips and that's the end of it. My favorite candy bar is a Snickers bar. You can get the fun size snickers bar, take half of it or cut it into quarters and let it melt into your mouth. I love to freeze them, so I put them in the freezer, and then you can crunch on them. Most over-eaters will literally eat a snickers bar in four bites, and it will be gone in a second.

I definitely feel like people who drink fruit juice, and it can be any kind of juice, apple juice, prune juice, grape juice, pineapple juice, may struggle because of the amount of sugar in the juice. I'm going to list a few different fruit juices here and I'm going to put the number of calories and the amount of sugar that I just googled for each of these.

Here is the information I pulled from Google.

Item	Grams of Sugar	Calories
½ Cup Strawberries	4g	98
1 Twizzler	5g	40
1 Mini Cannoli	6g	70
½ Cup Blueberries	7g	170
1 Reese's Cup	8g	87
1 Medium Chocolate Chip Cookie	9g	78
1 Fun Size Twix	9g	80
1 Cup Watermelon	10g	47
1 Krispy Cream Donut	10g	190
1 Medium Peach	13g	59
1 Slice Apple Pie	13g	67
1 Cup Cantaloupe	14g	60
1 Fudge Brownie	15g	110
10 (1oz) Gummy Bears	16g	87
1 Large Bannana	17g	121
1 Medium Pear	17g	105
1 Medium Apple	19g	105
1 Regular Size Payday Bar	21g	180
1 Slice Pumpkin Pie	25g	323
1 Slice Cheesecake	27g	401
1 Regular Size Snickers bar	27g	215
1 Slice of Birthday Cake	30g	424
1 Slice Pecan Pie	31g	117
1 King Size Milky Way	31g	230
1 Regular Size Skittles	45g	231

Juice - 8oz	Grams of Sugar	Calories
1 Cup Orange Juice	18g	103
1 Cup Apple Juice	27g	103
1 Cup Cranberry Juice	28g	105
1 Cup Pineapple Juice	32g	132
1 Cup Grape Juice	32g	136

So, one of the things that again, I'm seeing thin people do is when they have a dessert,

ONE MEAL TASTING AND A

they will only eat about 3/4 of a dessert every week or every other week. Let's say it was a piece of chocolate cake, they will eat maybe half or 3/4 of that piece of chocolate cake, maybe one a week or every other week. So in the end, they are eating maybe 400 calories worth of a dessert. This dessert is taking the place of another food meaning you're going to fill up to a level four and then eat all the way from a 4.0 and then end at 4.3 or 4.5.

Some of you, may choose approximately 50-75 calories per day as a meal finisher. What I like to do instead is just have a little bit of coffee with cream and then once every other week have 400 calories as one big dessert. I suggest doing this every other week if you want to be really thin. If you don't want to be super thin, then have one every week. I'm finding more about how little sugar they're having but again they're not depriving themselves.

In addition to not wanting to be overly stuffed during the day, they also consider whether or not the food they are presented with is really worth it. Recently I went to dinner with my friend Kellie. When we tasted the bread, she took one bite and she said, "it's not worth it." The bread didn't taste good enough to make it her grain and carb for the day. The next weekend we went to do a different restaurant. She took one bite of the bread and said, "This bread is worth every bite!" She meant that the carbs and calories in that bread was worth using her daily amount of carbs on those bites.

Let me give you another example: I have three pairs of shoes in my closet that are over $200 for each pair. But they were so gorgeous, I decided to buy them even though, in general, I don't spend more than $200 on a pair of shoes. It's a good example of something that I only do about once a year because those shoes are rare and worth the extra money. Most people are constantly aware of how much money they spend and how much they save. What if we thought about food in the same way? We must balance our checkbook or our Venmo account to keep track of what we spend. Just like we want to be financially wealthy, we want to be physically healthy. So, asking yourself similar questions when presented with food choices could totally impact your investment in your body over the long term. For example, for me, I love to go to Ritz Carlton and Four seasons. Every time I go, I spend too much money. Their massages are like $180 a pop. I also love to go to the spa, and I end up spending too much for the weekend. To make up for it when I get home, I don't buy any clothes, I don't buy new makeup, and I eat at home. This allows me to balance what I just spent. The same could (and should) be applied to how we eat.

So, how can you subscribe to the One Meal a Day (OMAD) concept and not feel *famished*? Initially, your body will take some time to adjust, especially if you've been eating a lot during the day. However, you'll get used to it, and you won't want to eat any other way. Remember: this is not a diet—diets don't work because they are not sustainable (remember, I've tried them *all!*). Rather, this is a change in the way you live in a relationship with food.

I am not big on depriving myself, but I love sugar. Even *I* can get out of control with sugar. Right now, we're all trying to boost our immune systems. Did you know that eating sugar can weaken your body's defenses significantly? Sugar feeds things like cancer cells and can cause the overgrowth of yeast in the body. Moreover, it can lead to diabetes and other conditions that can significantly impact your quality of life. Despite this, roughly 70 percent of Americans are eating way more sugar than they should have per day.

Your body gets its fuel from three kinds of food: carbohydrates, proteins, and fats. Carbohydrates (carbs) come from bread, fruits, vegetables, and more. Fat and protein come from meat, dairy, nuts, and fatty vegetables like avocados. Your digestive system breaks down each food and sends it to your digestive tract. Your body uses insulin to process the sugar from the carbs you eat. So, the amount of insulin your body creates really depends on how much sugar you're taking in. When you hear the word "sugar" you might be visualizing table sugar, but sugar also comes from the breakdown of carbs.

Just the other day I had one more interview with a super-skinny model. She eats all her daily calories in about a 4-hour eating window, just like so many of the other women I've talked to repeatedly, and she's very healthy. She will break her fast with a small meal at around 2 p.m. (when she feels a little hankering for something), then maybe a small snack at 4 p.m., and finally, a true dinner at around 6 p.m. Her dinner could be a green salad with half a cup of rice and some fresh grilled tuna while her midday snack maybe a couple of hard-boiled eggs or a small bit of grilled chicken. She follows the same pattern I've heard over and over again: vegetables with protein as the main staple of a day with about half a cup of grains and half a cup of fruit each day.

One of my friends at snack time, (let's say, around 1:00 p.m. or 2:00 p.m.) if she goes out to eat, she's getting a small side salad with very little dressing or she's having vegetables with hummus, basically a high protein snack with veggies. Sometimes she'll have a couple of hard-boiled eggs. Maybe she'll have some peanut butter with celery sticks or a turkey roll-up. A lot of times she'll have raw vegetables with some kind of mustard dressing that is very low in calories. Maybe she'll eat a sweet potato or a regular potato, but she'll have one serving of it and that's it. Mostly, she's having lots of veggies, like raw vegetables, and then for dinner, she eats whatever she wants—but she'll focus on high protein and high veggies.

OK, so let's say that you want to do One Meal a Day and a Tasting. Let's say you're on vacation and your breakfast is included with your meal. I don't do this when I'm at home, but while I'm on vacation I could have three eggs over medium. I don't eat the egg whites because of my sensitivity, so, I could eat three egg yolks for breakfast at around nine. And then at one o'clock, I could eat a salad with grilled chicken salad. And then I could skip dinner altogether. Maybe just drink coconut water.

Now I want to talk with you about being obsessed with food and dieting. One of the things that is really important is to make sure that I'm not thinking about food, reading about food, shopping for food prep, or constantly thinking about it all the time. I have to ask myself what I really want, like, what am I *really* wanting, and then I have to actually eat that. I do this because I know if I don't then I'm going to crave something else and then I'm going to eat more. I need to make sure that I eat what I really want, what I'm really craving, and get exactly that. My son is a perfect example of this: if he doesn't absolutely love something we give him to eat, then he just won't eat it. I have seen it over and over again, with my thin friends and it is so important.

I want to share another story with you- One of my friends got a grilled chicken salad that was really plain because it was healthy, and I got chicken fajitas which I love. She really wanted the chicken fajitas but decided against it. I ended up eating about a third of the fajitas, but she ate her salad *and* the rest of my fajitas because she was not satisfied. So be careful! You really need to balance it.

You will hear a similar version of this story again later in this book. It is intentional that I repeat myself and say things over again in this book. I say things multiple times for you to truly internalize it. One of my friends, Michelle, read my first book and lost five pounds, but then was stuck at a plateau. I told her go back and listen to my audiobook three times. She listened to it every day for 15 minutes a day, and guess what? She lost her last 15 pounds. The more times you hear this truth, the more successful you will be.

There is this Italian restaurant here called *Aldo's* and they have this dish called "Shrimp Gorgonzola". It is *so* good! You can get just the shrimp as an appetizer and get it without the pasta, which is what I normally do. Guess what? That totally satisfies me! I could get the pasta and get my satisfied meter to a 9 or 10, but I was just as satisfied with just the shrimp.

Let's talk about hunger and fullness. You have to get in tune with your body and ask, "How hungry am I? How full am I?" This is the only way you're going to successfully lose weight with intermittent fasting. When you learn how to evaluate **true hunger**, you're going to discover you don't need to eat as much food or as many meals as you think. My experience with the thinnest women I met with: they eat either one meal or one meal and a tasting. The time they only have one meal is when they go out to eat and have had a lot of food and got their fullness scale to a 4 or 4.1, which sustains them for the full day.

Take the story of sisters Edna and Nona. They decided they were going to eat the exact same thing. Edna decided even though she committed to eating the same thing as Nona, that she wanted to have a little something for breakfast. Nona ate nothing for breakfast, lost three almost four pounds that week, but everything else they ate was the same for lunch and dinner. Edna had the audacity to say, "I knew I wasn't going to lose weight eating the tacos and the fajitas I ate this week." The sister who lost weight ate the same thing. I asked her why she ate the hard-boiled egg and toast for breakfast, and she said she thought she had to eat something in the morning to start the day. Her response was the one boiled egg only had about 80 calories, and half a piece of sprouted grain toast had 50 calories, plus a little bit of butter, so it was between 150-200 calories and she didn't think it was that big of a deal. It *was* a big deal because Nona had lost the full 3½ – 4lbs because she didn't have those things for breakfast.

This is the most profound sentence: say this sentence to yourself, "eating any food, even if you think it's super healthy or it's low calorie when you're not physically hungry will cause you to put on weight." Learning and understanding your hunger scale is one of the most important things that you can do for yourself and your weight loss journey. Like my friend Catherine says, "I love when I'm hungry! I love when I hear my stomach growl because when I hear my stomach growl and when I get hungry, I know my body is eating its own fat."

Let me give you an example of the balance of eating healthy and getting the results you want. This is how I eat chips and guacamole at a Mexican restaurant. I love guacamole, but I have to be careful because I can tend to eat too much of it. What I do is, I get the guacamole, but I always have people with me so I always share. I take the guacamole and put a couple spoonfuls on my plate and that's all I'm going to allow myself to have. Often, I ask if they have cucumbers and if they can slice some up for me. I eat them with the guacamole and then I might take two maybe four chips and I eat that with the guacamole with some salsa. I love the cucumber, so I don't feel deprived when I eat them, they are crunchy, and I love it. Sometimes I want a little more crunch, so I will eat a couple of chips, but not too many.

As I was interviewing people, I noticed that there were two kinds of eaters. Some people were sweets people, and some people are salty people. Then some people love crunchy foods and some people love soft foods

For me, there is no question that I have a serious sweet tooth. I have always loved chocolate, soft moist cake, crunchy cookies, ice cream, and all types of candy. While I definitely have my moments craving chips or pizza, my sweet tooth outweighs my salty cravings all day long.

Each one of the thin eater's I interviewed said they either craved crunchy or a creamy soft food. I will list some examples of each; see which one you identify with more.

Crunchy Foods

Carrots, chips, hard tacos, crispy cookies, the outside of the brownie, hard cheddar cheese, brownie brittle, crispy fries, crunchy peanuts

SoftFoods

Cooked veggies, soft tacos, soft cookies, the middle of the brownie, whipped cream cheese, soft warm chocolate cake, mashed potatoes, creamy peanut butter.

Which sounds more like you? It is important to find out if you're crunchy or soft, sweet or salty, so that you can make sure that you are able to get some of these elements in your meal. Otherwise, you will tend to over eat and not be satisfied.

I personally am a sweet and crunchy girl! My husband is a soft and sweet combination. There is no right or wrong category for you to be! Every person has a target of where they have their satiety center. Pretend that you have a target to hit, and in the bull's-eye is a smile. When you hit the bull's-eye, that makes you smile. When you enjoy the food that satisfies your soft or crunchy side, or your salty or sweet side, you have hit your happy target! In my day, I usually have about half a cup of berries or half a cup of pomegranate. Other salty loving thin eaters might need to have half a cup of chips, or half a cup of salted pistachios.

One of the most important things that you are going to do is learn to make sure that you eat at either a level one or level zero on the hunger scale or what I like to call "Hungry, Hungry Hippo" level. What is a hungry, hungry hippo? In my first edition of my book, I called it "Hamster Hungry" because I had a friend who went out of town and when she came back, she realized her hamster had eaten all its babies because it ran out of food!

But once they knew the origin of the story, people were like "Eww gross! I don't want to call it hamster hungry after that," so I changed it to Hungry, Hungry Hippo.

Let's look at the levels of hunger, which we will go over in more detail later.

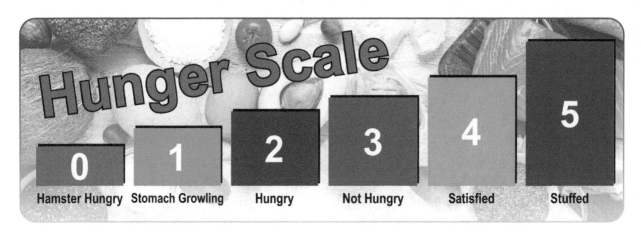

Hunger Scale

| 0 | 1 | 2 | 3 | 4 | 5 |
| Hamster Hungry | Stomach Growling | Hungry | Not Hungry | Satisfied | Stuffed |

Level 0: Starving, ravenous, grouchy, weak, all you can think about is what to eat and how to get it.

Level 1: Your stomach is growling, and you feel completely on E. You can physically hear your stomach growl. 95 % of people do hear their stomach growl when hungry although there are about 5% that do not. Make sure when at level 1 your stomach is growling because it is empty and not just digesting food from a previous meal. Everything sounds good to eat at this level.

Level 2: Hungry, starting to think about what sounds good to you. You are deciding what your body is craving.

Level 3: You are not hungry but not really full either. Kind of neutral.

Level 4: You are satisfied. This is where you want to end all of your meals.

Level 5: Stuffed, uncomfortably full. You don't want to let it get to that point.

You should always eat to a 3.8 to 3.9 or a level 4.

Even though I say in the book you are going to have one meal and a tasting, that can be breakfast/lunch or lunch/dinner for your tasting. One of the easiest meals to give up is breakfast. I'd like for you to try this when you're starting: go the longest that you can in the day without eating breakfast, and then go as long as you can without eating lunch and then have your first tasting. You may be thinking to yourself, "I can't do that! Breakfast is too important I can't handle not eating breakfast!" This is a lie from the devil saying that if we don't have a little something in the morning, we won't be able to have a great day; that you won't have the stamina for the day. If you're not hungry you shouldn't be eating something. Now as you get more advanced, I'd like to change things up and instead of eating lunch and dinner, you do breakfast and lunch. I will say out of all the women I interviewed almost all of them did a tasting around 2 p.m. or 3 p.m. and then they ate again at 6 p.m. or 7 p.m.

Remember - you are not taking one bite of food until you are sure that you have reached level zero or one. Some people get there at 11 o'clock, some people get there at 12 o'clock, but I will tell you the thinnest women I interview will have their coffee with a little bit of cream or black coffee and they wait until around 2 o'clock to have their first tasting. If you can push it that long, go ahead and do it. If you can't, make sure your body is at a level 0 or 1 and go from there.

One of the things my friend Catherine always says (who was Miss Virginia and has a perfect body), is that she loves the idea of being hungry. She gets excited to be hungry; being hungry is not the end of the world. People will say "Oh I am hungry," GREAT! You have to change your mindset to "it is the best thing ever that I'm hungry."

My friend Kristin's husband kept nagging her about how important breakfast was. She has never had a weight problem and has always been thin. She started having a smoothie every morning because her husband was making his and kept saying, "You should be having a smoothie in the morning." Even though she wasn't hungry, she decided to try it and she gained about five pounds in a month. First of all, the thing with smoothies is you have to be careful. Smoothies can have a lot of calories depending on what you put in them. One smoothie can have anywhere from 400 to 600 calories! The main thing for Kristin wasn't the calories, it was that she was now eating breakfast when she wasn't hungry. She wasn't doing intermittent fasting, and of course, she's going to gain that weight. She was now eating breakfast, lunch, and dinner *and* having a smoothie when she wasn't hungry because she listened to her husband. He said, "well you really should have something in the morning" and boom she gained five pounds in less than 30 days.

I have a friend who owns a farm, and she says that her farmworkers start working around 4 a.m. and they end up eating around 9 a.m. Of course, they're hungry at 9 a.m. because they've already put in five hours of work. Let's say you wake up at 7 a.m. and maybe you work out. I work out every morning on an empty stomach and in a fasted state. So, let say you get to work at 9 a.m. and five hours later that is around 1 o'clock, you're going to be hungry. So again, it depends on when are you starting your day. Now for me, I usually do get up around 4 or 5 a.m. so it depends, but sometimes I'll eat around noon, and sometimes I will try to wait until 2 p.m.

One of the other most important things for you to do, (that I am terrible at and I am not even going to lie about), is slow down when you eat. I even talk about this in my book *Waist Away*, it is such a struggle for me. I watch my thin eaters and how well they do with eating slowly. It turns out that taking our time to enjoy a meal actually does make it taste better. Our mouths are structured to allow us to get a strong whiff of our food's aroma, which enhances how we perceive its flavor, but only if we breathe slowly and quietly. We may miss out on this enhanced experience if we scarf down our meals.

We have over 10,000 taste buds in our mouths. I love to take big bites and literally swallow before I even taste anything. I don't know what it is or why I do this, but I have trained myself to do it, so I literally have to un-train myself to not do this. This is going to be one of the most painful things you are going to do, but it really helps. I take a couple of bites of food and push it away, and then have a couple more bites and push it away, and in between eating I may take a 5–10-minute break in-between. Sometimes I say I am full or sometimes I decide to eat a few more bites.

How many people do you know that eat one pistachio and then put it down, then get another one? Most people will take tons at a time. One of the things that I can get out of control with is nuts, I would literally eat like a cup and a half of nuts, (which is really way too much too many calories) and you just don't need that much. One of my favorite foods is pistachios. I try to get the pistachios that are already shelled. I would literally take a whole mini package, open it and put half of it in my mouth, and then take the other half and eat it. Before I know it, I've finished the entire mini bag of pistachios. Now I try to get the pistachios that I have to shell myself - I open one up, put it in my mouth hoping that I found a salty one. I take my time and look for one that is easier to open, put one nut in my mouth, and slowly chew it to make sure I experience the taste and flavor. I have to remind myself all the time that there are no teeth in my stomach! I have to make my food literally melt and mush before I swallow.

Now there are two tricks that I want to make sure that you do for eating slowly. Number one is to set a timer for 25 minutes for your meal. Once you try this, you are going to say there is no way (unless you're already a slow eater) that I can do this. Setting a timer is the only way that I can do this. I learned this from my friend Catherine, and she will say, "You can do it, too." After about 10 minutes of eating, she literally takes a break from the food and pushes it away. It's so hysterical because I've gone out to eat with her several times and every time the waiter comes by at least three or four times and says are you finished eating that and she says no. The way she kind of pushes it away and sits back in her seat and puts her fork down so it looks like she's done and then she'll eat a couple more bites and then she'll push it away again and then the waiter will come by again and will be like, "OK, can I take that?" and she's like, "no, I'm not finished yet." Usually, it's not until the fourth time, (and it has been about 25 minutes or longer) they come by that she says "yes." The reason she says that she does this is because it takes about 25 minutes for your body to register that you're full and that you're satiated.

Number two is to understand that being full is not the same as being satiated. This is so important! I shared the story of my friend Ali in my book *Waist Away*. We went to *Uno's* for an event once. I never eat pizza, but I decided to get a small personal one. She decided on the grilled chicken as a healthier option. After she was done with the salad, she asked me if I was going to finish mine and then proceeded to eat the rest of my pizza. She really wanted the pizza but chose the salad since she thought it was healthier and she wasn't satisfied. I always try to pick a healthy option, but if I really want pizza, I might get a cauliflower crust pizza or something like that, so I will be satisfied. If I want Mexican food, I'm going to get Mexican food. I might pick a healthier option, but if I really want something, I'll have a couple of bites and be done with it.

The other really important thing is that you don't drink during your meals. You want to drink outside of your meals, and you want to keep yourselves hydrated, but you do not want to drink anything while you're eating a meal. This is going to be very difficult for you, but you'll going to learn how to do this.

Remember:

Those of you who have food issues, the devil will use these lies over and over:

- Breakfast is the most important meal of the day; it will make sure that you have enough energy for the day.
- I've always heard I should eat three meals a day or I should clean my plate because there are starving kids in China.
- I should always save the best for last.
- I've heard that if you skip meals that you will end up gaining more weight. If you don't eat enough food your body will go into starvation mode.
- I need some sugar so that it'll give me a quick boost of energy.

If you've read my prior books, *Fasting to Freedom*, *Waist Away the Chantel Ray Way*, and *Freedom from Food Bible Study Workbook*, you know I've been on quite a journey with my weight loss efforts!

I used to say things like:

- ✔ I'm never eating again.
- ✔ I would be happier if I were thinner.
- ✔ I'm going on a diet on Monday.
- ✔ I look at food and it goes to my hips.
- ✔ I wonder how she eats like that and stays so thin?
- ✔ How does she eat all that food and still have a perfect body?
- ✔ This will never work for me; I will just gain it right back.

However, after I interviewed so many women, I realized that many of them never dieted and yet they always stayed the same size! But *how* did they do it? The principles outlined in this book will explain just that and so much more.

First things first: Taste is very important to me and to all the thin women that I have interviewed! Fad diets will encourage you to eat foods that are bland and unenjoyable. Who wants to do that?! Everyone wants to enjoy and savor the food they eat, regardless of your weight loss or maintenance goals. Based on my discussions with women who maintain their weight naturally, this is entirely possible to do.

As I interviewed other thin women, I realized that they ate what I call a "Keto flex diet". Most of them couldn't put a name on it if you asked them, but the trends among them remained the same. They would eat mostly vegetables, moderate protein and, healthy fats. They kept servings of grain to a minimum and ate fruit sparingly. Instead of agonizing over their food choices, they became really good at listening to their bodies to determine what to eat. As you read this book, you will learn how to get in tune with your body and your individual needs so that you can finally break free from the cycle of dead-end dieting and enjoy food again! Additionally, I've included easy recipes for meals or "tastings" to help guide you along the way.

ONE MEAL A DAY (OMAD)

Of the women I interviewed, 10% of them ate "one meal a day", or what I will refer to as "OMAD" for the rest of the book. Even though 70% ate two meals, for a lot of them, it was more like one meal and a "tasting". You may think eating OMAD sounds absolutely ridiculous, but it actually can save you a ton of time and money. Once your body gets used to it, it's not nearly as hard as it sounds. When I am in a maintenance mode, I like to eat in a six-hour window, but when I have gained a few pounds and really want to lose weight, eating in a one-hour eating window and eating OMAD is what really works for shedding those extra pounds.

OMAD is based on the principles of intermittent fasting. In my opinion, the reason intermittent fasting is so effective is because you are always in a fed state or a fasted state. The only way you could eat something while your body would still think you are in a fasted state is if you just ate straight fat. So, if you ate just a tablespoon of ghee, your body would still think you were in a fasted state. As soon as your body starts digesting all the nutrients from whatever you ate, and for several hours after, depending on the food you ate, your body is basically creating insulin. When it creates insulin, the insulin signals your body to store the food it has taken in. Your body has a choice: it can take the food in as body fat or as glycogen. If your glycogen stores are totally full already because you are not hungry and have enough already stored up, then your body is not ever-burning fat, because it is in complete storage mode. If I drink MCT oil or coconut oil with my coffee, it can cause me to gain weight. My body can choose the fat I gave it or the fat on my hips. I rather my body eat my fat from my hips or stomach.

What does that hour of OMAD look like for me? For a while, I started eating my OMAD at lunch, which I like doing, but I have so much more energy, and I am so much more productive during the day when I don't eat. Instead of eating something quick for lunch, I really enjoy that OMAD at dinner with my family. When I was doing the OMAD at lunch, I sat down at the dinner table one night to actually eat, and my son, who always sets the table, put just a glass of water in front of me. I said, "Hun, I'm eating dinner tonight," and he was so shocked because it had been so long since I had actually eaten dinner with them! I switched my OMAD to dinner. The thing that works the best is for me to have a very small tasting around 2pm and dinner with my family.

If I choose to eat OMAD for the day, the very first thing I do in that hour is usually eat some sort of high-fat food. I am usually very hungry after 23 hours, and this helps calm my body down and ease into digestion. I might have a quarter of avocado or some almonds— just a small amount of fat because it helps fill me up. It is almost like an appetizer. If I am

ONE MEAL AND A TASTING

out to dinner, I will order chicken lettuce wraps or something similar so that I can be a little bit fuller; then I eat my meal. If I am going to have a dessert, I will wait a bit and have a little dessert. But let's be clear - even though I am having dessert, I am not eating a huge slice of cheesecake! Instead, I would eat some berries with whipped cream. This would satisfy that sweet tooth without causing pain, discomfort, or regret. If this is your first time trying OMAD, I don't suggest that you go from eating three or four meals a day to just one meal a day. It's great if you decide you're going to start intermittent fasting, starting with an 8-hour window, then a 6-hour window, then a 4-hour window and work your way down.

You must decide how and when you do best with your OMAD. Only you know how your body feels when you eat certain foods. Remember most of the thin eaters do OMAD and a tasting, not just OMAD. It is up to you to determine when is the best time to consume your food for the day. Some people prefer to eat all of their daily required calories at breakfast time, some at lunch, and some at dinner. I only know one person who eats mostly breakfast and doesn't really eat lunch or dinner. There are many different viewpoints out there, and there is no absolute right answer to what is best. In my opinion, if you want to work with your body as much as possible, eating later in the day is preferred. I just feel like I am so much more productive during the day with the number of things I can get done when I don't eat.

Our bodies spend much of the day under the control of the sympathetic branch of our nervous system. This system controls the fight or flight response and helps us respond and react to stress. During the day, our bodies are naturally a little more stressed. As the day goes on and we transition into night, the parasympathetic branch of the nervous system kicks in. I talked about this earlier. This branch promotes rest and digestion. In the latter part of the day, our bodies are better suited for good digestion. I would say more than 90% of the people I know use dinner, or they eat what they call linner (late lunch with a dinner), as their OMAD. They will have their tasting usually around 1 pm to 2 pm. Eating later in the day also makes it convenient to enjoy your meals with friends. You can still participate in family dinners around the dining room table, go to a dinner party, or join friends out for an evening meal.

Recently, I went to a fancy French lunch with friends to celebrate a birthday. We arrived at 1:00 p.m., but by the time we ate, it was 2:00 p.m. Because it was a big lunch in the middle of the day, that was the only meal for me and some of my friends for the whole day. If your meal satisfies your nutritional needs for the day and satisfies your hunger, there is no need to eat anything other than that meal. I cannot stress enough that the more interviews I do, the more people I find who are doing some kind of snack around

2 o'clock and then eating dinner. But if they know they're going out for a big party, they might not have anything at all for lunch and save it all for that dinner. On the days that you have a bigger lunch, and you weren't hungry for dinner, you could either sit and enjoy the company while having nothing to eat or perhaps order a side of vegetables or a small salad so that you're not the ONLY one at the table not eating. However, my friends and I have gone to lunch countless times where one or more of us have not eaten because we were not hungry.

One of the things that really helps people wait until 2 o'clock to eat is having coffee with almond milk, coconut milk, MCT oil, or cream. I always like to say that it's best if you can train your body to have black coffee, but most of the people I interview say they have coffee with cream in the morning, which allows them to wait until 2 o'clock to eat their first tasting. You can time your meals based on what works for you, not what others prefer. We eat a very early dinner in my family. I had a girl call me at 4:45 p.m. one time, and she said, "What are you doing?" I said, "Oh I'm finishing dinner." She was surprised and was like "At 4:45?!" You *can* eat an earlier dinner; you don't have to wait until 7:00. I feel like the nice thing also is that at the end of the day, I'm more relaxed, and my digestion in the later part of the day is better. I can take my time; I'm not worried about work or other things, and I can slow down a little bit. Just remember that even if you decide to eat a big meal at lunchtime, there's no reason you can't participate in a family dinner or go to a dinner party because you don't *have* to eat to enjoy the experience. That is the biggest thing: people who are thin feel no pressure to eat just because they are at a dinner or function. A lot of times, I'll go to different lunch meetings or parties, and people will say, "Oh, eat something small," but I'll sit there and not eat. You must get out of your mind that you have to eat just because you've been invited to an event or party. Eating has nothing to do with enjoying someone's company … NOTHING. In fact, not eating actually makes the time more meaningful because you aren't shoving food in your face, and you can talk more.

When you're eating one full meal, eat whatever you want, however, when I watch the thin eaters eat, they maybe had a small serving of grains or a small serving of fruit. It's ideal to have vegetables and a protein as the major components of that meal, but eat what you want, eat what you're craving. If you want a steak, eat a steak. If you want chicken, eat chicken. Whatever it is that your body craves at that time, go for it.

Let me tell you some reasons why I love doing OMAD and a tasting lifestyle:

- **It Saves You Money**

  You will actually save money. If I'm not saving money, it's because I'm eating really healthy, clean food for that one meal. I might pick something up from somewhere, and it might be a 30-dollar meal. Some people spend $10 on breakfast, lunch, and dinner all the time, but I choose to spend $30 collectively on one single meal and get way better food. You can either save money and eat a $10 meal or get something more expensive and of higher quality.

- **It Improves Digestion**

  When you fast for so long, it gives all of your systems a way to rest. It can give your pancreas, your gallbladder, and other organs a rest. It can really help people who have IBS and like issues.

- **It Helps You Stop Thinking About Food**

  The weird thing is, when I put in my mind that I'm not eating for that whole day, I literally do not think about food. I can focus on other things. You might think that if you're only eating once a day, you're going to be ravenous! But when your body transitions from a sugar-burning mode to a fat-burning mode, you are less hungry. If you are ravenous that is why a tasting is so important. It helps you not be crazy hungry.

- **It Increases Energy**

  I'm telling you when I eat OMAD, I just feel lighter and bubblier. The amount I can accomplish is just so much more when food isn't weighing me down. Another reason I like eating dinner instead of lunch is that I avoid the three o'clock slump. People are generally finishing their lunch around one or two o'clock, and that is when they start getting tired and sluggish, and their blood sugar starts dropping. I avoid that when I eat OMAD at dinner.

- **It Decreases Inflammation**

  I have a lot of issues with joint pain and inflammation; my knees swell up and my joints hurt. But when I am doing OMAD and a tasting, really making sure that the food is of high quality for that one meal, it really helps with these issues.

- **It Saves Calories**

I don't count calories, but I know just from the amount of food that I'm eating that I don't eat as many calories in one meal as I would be eating three meals in a day. Some days, when I am eating just one meal, I eat more than other days, which is natural. But often, because I haven't eaten all day, I get full really quickly, so my portion sizes are smaller. If you're listening to your hunger and your satiety signals when eating OMAD, you're going to eat less food. In the beginning, because they are waiting all day to eat, some people over-eat. You must make sure you are still eating to the point right before you're full and *not* passing that point. If you are interested in going on an extended fast, then you need to get my book *Fasting to Freedom*. The guidance in that book is different than if you are just going to do OMAD because the fasting period is longer.

Most experts agree as for **having coffee** or tea during **your** fast — **you** should be just fine. Some experts say , **if you drink** coffee with less than 50 calories, then **your** body **will** remain in **the fasted**state. So, **your coffee** with **a** splash of milk or **cream** is just fine. Others will say absolutely not!

I also personally believe Caffiene also has a stronger effect when ingested on an empty stomach, so it does a better job at helping you battle fatigue and "brain fog." This makes increased concentration another perk of intermittent fasting with coffee.

Technically, you're not fasting if you add any of these to your coffee because they all contain calories. However, fats themselves won't influence your insulin or blood sugar levels, so some experts say this is the most-recommended choice if you're looking to boost your insulin sensitivity , if you have prediabetes or diabetes

While you may have heard recommendations for "bulletproof coffee"--made by adding butter , coconut oil and MCT oil to coffee--be aware that it contains over 230 calories in a 16-ounce serving (made with a tablespoon of each fat). So you are adding tons of fat and calories

I want to say that 90% of the women that I interviewed did have a splash of cream in the coffee with no sugar because they just didn't like the taste and most of them had half-and-half organic or fresh cream. So on the other hand, I have seen people who have taken cream out of their diet and lost that extra 10 pounds they needed to lose just from taking the cream out of the coffee. This is something you have to decide but I wanted to make clear that the people who were thin, 90% did put a splash of cream in their coffee. Remember you can train your body to have black tea or black coffee or green tea with no cream. Another option is to break your fast around noon and have coffee with cream then.

For me what I do is I have a cup or 2 of green tea in the morning, and then around 12pm I'll have a cup of coffee with a splash of cream. I have trained my body to not like sugar in my tea or coffee. I know tons of people who have trained themselves to like coffee completely black, I drink black coffee sometimes.

I would rather wait until noon to have a cup of coffee with cream because I like that more and that takes me to about 2pm to eat my first tasting! I said, I know a lot to thin women who have a splash of cream in their coffee and thrill are still super thin.

THINGS YOU CAN HAVE FASTING WITH OMAD:

Great
Water
Black coffee
Tea unflavored with no added flavors or sweeteners
Herbal tea unflavored and not fruity
Unflavored sparkling water like San Pellegrino, Perrier, and La Croix

Crutch Drinks, if you absolutely need a crutch! (However, try to have no oil or cream at all.)
MCT (medium-chain triglycerides) Oil
Coconut oil
Ghee
Heavy Cream (if not allergic to dairy)
(These are all crunch drink options to add to your coffee if you need to have a creamer.) I have seen some people lose tons of weight by adding these to their coffee. It also stumps a lot of people in their weight loss. This a crutch drink, and ultimately you want to get off the crutches.

Also, crutch items but okay
Organic Stevia
Regular Creamer (unsweetened)
Coconut Milk
Almond Milk (to make it at home, see my video at <u>chantelrayway.com/recipes</u>)
Homemade bone broth—*I use this for extended fasting, but if you are just fasting for 23 hours, you should be fine. If you need to use this as a crutch in the very beginning that's okay but only for a couple of days to help you. You shouldn't need it continuously, and at the max have one cup.*

Absolutely Not
Artificial sweeteners
Saccharine
NutraSweet
Aspartame

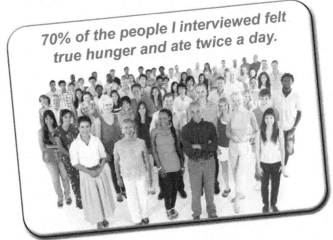

70% of the people I interviewed felt true hunger and ate twice a day.

WHAT IS A "TASTING?"

As I mentioned, perpetually thin women choose to have some sort of snack during their eating window, which is usually no more than about 200-400 calories. And, again, they don't *count* those calories, they just choose things that satisfy, without being equal to a meal. So, what would a tasting like that consist of? What's left over from yesterday's meal? Did you put a small leftover in the fridge that would make a good tasting?

A "tasting" is the equivalent of a snack. The size of the tasting depends on the individual. Some of the people who were thin might have calorie tasting that would amount to 150 – 250 calories. This could be a protein bar or a handful of almonds or vegetables and hummus. The tasting is most of the time whatever their body is craving. For example, my friend Laurie may have a healthy Starbucks protein bar because it's quick and easy to eat on the run. My friend Kellie, however, will have raw veggies and a little bit of hummus with maybe one slice of turkey.

Some examples of tastings you can try are:

- Carrot chips with honey mustard and feta cheese, half of an apple, and 2 pieces of turkey.
- Leftover salad from the night before, basic salad with feta cheese with a honey mustard dressing with 2 slices of deli turkey.
- Red peppers and celery with ½ cup of strawberries or ½ cup of cantaloupe.
- 1 slice of Cauliflower pizza.

Let's talk about what I referred to as hunger snacks in my book *Waist Away.* As I interviewed different women, almost all of them had a solution for curbing their appetites before it was time to eat. I asked, "When you're hungry, what do you do to keep yourself from binging and keep yourself from getting so ravenously hungry?" All of them said that they either use a hunger drink or a hunger snack. One of the things that my mom and aunt used to say to me all the time was, "Slow down!" I would get myself to the point that I was so hungry that once I would eat *all* of the food in front of me and I would eat too fast!

If you look in my mom's purse at any given time, she always has snacks in her bag: raw or dry roasted almonds with no oil, walnuts, or cashews. And usually, when you are in the car with her, within 30 minutes to an hour before lunch, she pulls out her bag of walnuts, and she has each kind of snack in different little Ziploc bags. She has almonds in one bag, walnuts in another bag, and she literally pulls out each bag and says, "Who wants walnuts?" "Who wants almonds?" She sounds almost like the people at the baseball games selling the snacks in the stands or the people at the carnival who say, "Peanuts! Soda! Popcorn!"

I would say a good 50% of the people I interviewed carry some sort of hunger snack with them at all times. Nuts, fruit, or dried fiber cereal are the top three things that people say they carry with them. It varied, but nuts were the number one thing that people carried. This is likely because they are high in fat and provide quick satiety. Kim carries Crackling Oat Bran cereal with her at all times in a little snack baggie or some kind of fruit. Some might bring a little bag of carrots, but they almost always would eat some sort of snack about 30 minutes to an hour before they were going to eat, so they wouldn't be ravenously hungry.

Hunger snacks can only be consumed inside your eating window. They're meant to be high-protein, high-fat snacks that keep you from feeling ravenous. The best hunger snacks you can pick are nuts, like cashews or almonds. If you can't find something high in fat, then look for a high-fiber food. Good options are an apple with peanut butter, half of an avocado, a pickle, or an egg. Don't make your hunger snack a processed, high-carb food.

Time Open/Closed Eating Window	Level of Hunger	Meal or Tasting	Before Picture	After Picture
1pm	0	Tasting		
5pm	1	Meal		

Two Tastings and a Meal

Sometimes one tasting isn't enough to get you through the day, so you may add another one to help you as you near your OMAD. A lot of people lean towards this model in the winter months when temperatures drop, and our activity levels decrease. Our bodies tend to crave more food in the winter to deal with the dip in temperature, while the opposite happens in the summer (hello bikini season!). When the heat rises outside, most people naturally resort to a small taste of something, perhaps some fruit or nuts, and one substantial meal a day. This allows them to be focused and satiated, but not overly full.

This way of eating is really about making the choices that work for you, but not obsessing over the details. If you wake up and crave a hearty breakfast, that caloric load should be able to sustain you for much of the day, with a grazing of food here and there. Most of my friends, however, prefer to jumpstart their day with a cup of coffee (sans cream, mind you!) and have a larger meal later in the day when they've used up their energy stores. Plus, as I'm sure you can tell, our prime time is dinner. I've enjoyed hundreds of dinners with these women and know that this is the time that we can all really enjoy our food and perhaps a fun-size treat for dessert.

Time Open/Closed Eating Window	Level of Hunger	Meal or Tasting	Before Picture	After Picture
11am	0	Tasting	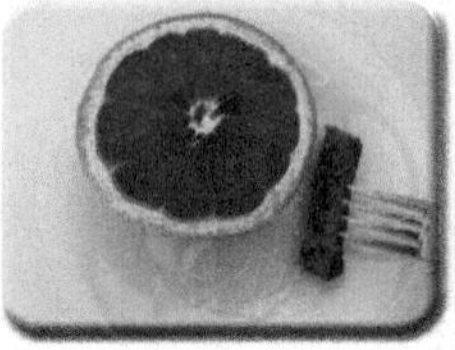	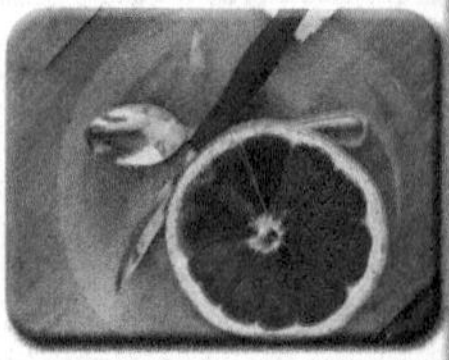
2pm	2	Meal	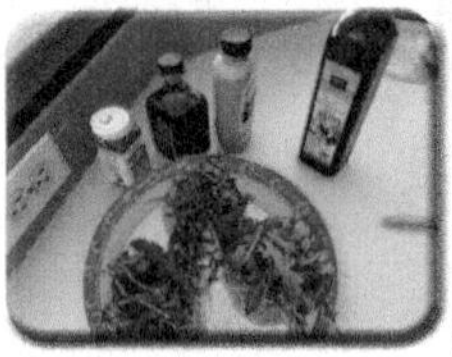	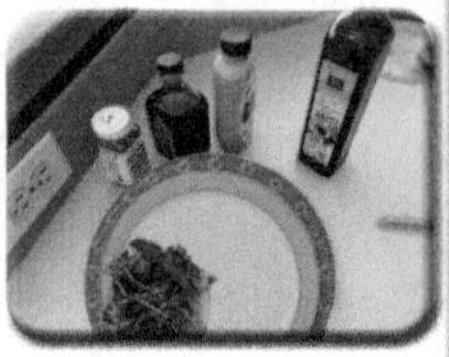
5pm	1	Tasting	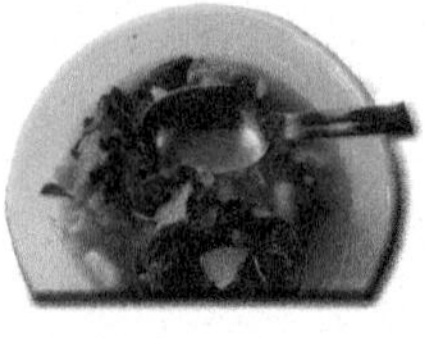	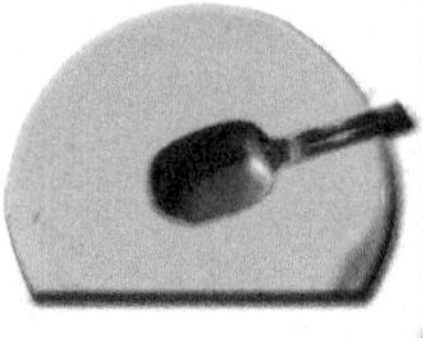

ONE MEAL AND A TASTING

32

If you've read my prior books, *Fasting to Freedom*, *Waist Away the Chantel Ray Way*, and *Freedom from Food Bible Study Workbook*, you know that I promote intermittent fasting as not only the best way to *lose* unwanted weight but also as the best way to keep it off for good and stay healthy. I first heard about intermittent fasting from my trainer, Chris Sykes. He lost 20 pounds in two weeks, and we had a mutual friend who lost 30 pounds in 60 days. Chris explained to me that I could eat whatever I wanted, all I had to do was confine myself to an eight-hour eating window. I thought that didn't sound too hard as I was already used to eating nine hours a day, even though I didn't know it at the time. After two weeks of trying the eight-hour window, I didn't lose any weight. I realized that cutting my eating down by one hour wasn't having an effect on me. So, I decided to reduce my eating window to six hours. By the third week, I lost 6 pounds in total.

Let's begin with a refresher on intermittent fasting from my book *Waist Away the Chantel Ray Way*. **Intermittent fasting** is a cycle of eating where you select what is called an **eating window** of time to eat and then fast for the rest. The most common window is called 16:8 – you fast for 16 hours and eat within an 8-hour window. This doesn't mean that you eat for the ENTIRE eight hours! Rather, you continue to make conscious food choices, but once that window closes, you're done for the day. In my research, I interviewed over 1,000 thin people and most of them did not have a **specific hour** of the day that they ate (e.g., lunch at 12, dinner at 6). They all ate *naturally* based on when they were actually hungry. I would ask someone, "What do you eat and what time do you eat?" Nine times out of ten they would say, "You know, I'm just not a big breakfast person. I never eat breakfast, so I start eating around 1 o'clock and then I usually eat dinner around 5:30 p.m. I pretty much finish around 6:00 p.m." I would ask another person, and she would say, "I start eating a snack around 2:00 p.m., I'll have something small, and then I will have dinner around 6:30 p.m." After interviewing them more in-depth, I realized that all of them were eating one medium-size meal and a snack or "tasting". For example, my friend Laura owns a marketing company and is always on the run. When I asked her, "what did you eat yesterday?" she remarked that she had a big lunch and said, "you know I was full, so I didn't eat anything the rest of the day!" This is a perfect example of how I would have watched her eat that big meal and in the past, I would have said, "See, she can eat whatever she wants and still stay so thin!" But before, I didn't realize that's all she ate the whole day. I would eat exactly what she ate but then go home and eat dinner, and be like "Why am I not thin? I ate exactly what she did!" When in reality, I had eaten so much more.

You open your eating window when you consume your very first meal, snack, or caloric drink of the day. You close your eating window after you consume your very last calorie. When you're fasting, you can only drink water, coffee, or unsweetened tea. There is no magic number of hours that every person should use for their eating window. Eight hours works great for some and six hours is better for others. Be mindful regardless if you have an eight hour or six-hour eating window, that you don't spend it consuming as many calories as you can by filling up on unhealthy food. You still have to obey the rules of hunger and eating healthy. The length of your eating window should be what works best for you with consideration to the portion sizes you eat.

The basis of this lifestyle is this: you don't restrict *what* you eat, but *when* you eat. You can eat what you like when you are physically hungry, as long as you only eat in your eating window and follow the FIRES Principles that were introduced in *Waist Away*:

Fast on a regular basis.

Identify true hunger.

Reduce sugar and white, simple carbohydrates.

Enjoy real food without deprivation.

Stop before you're full.

These Principles work together with intermittent fasting. If you think you can lose weight by eating non-stop for eight hours straight, then you're sadly mistaken! FIRES will help you to **never overeat** and to **eat only when you're truly hungry.**

Below is a chart with examples of sample eating windows:

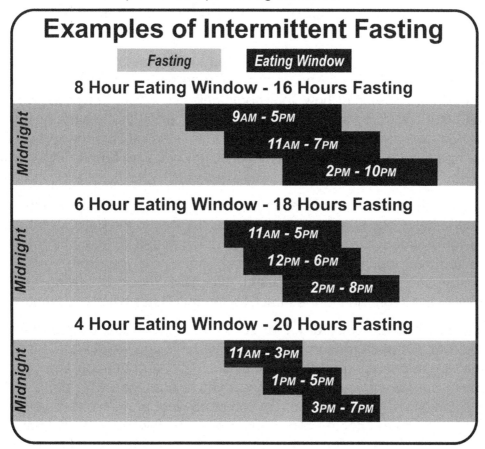

If you're eating window is eight hours long, then that means you're fasting for 16 hours. If you're eating for six hours, then you're fasting for 18. This is also called the **clock approach** as seen in the image below.

4 Hour Eating Window	6 Hour Eating Window	8 Hour Eating Window
2-6pm, 3-7pm, 4-8pm	3-9pm,2-8pm, 1-7pm	1-9pm,2-10pm, 3-11pm

When using the clock approach, I recommend starting with an eight-hour window while following the FIRES Principles. If you don't see yourself losing weight, start reducing your window. As you can see from the chart, if I'm doing the **20-hour fast**, then I'm only eating from 2 p.m. – 6 p.m., 3 p.m. – 7 p.m., or 4 p.m. – 8 p.m. I'm fasting the rest of the time. With the six-hour window, I'm eating from 3 p.m. - 9 p.m. and, again, fasting the rest of the time. The beauty of this approach is that you get to choose the window of when you want to eat that works with your schedule. I have tons of friends who like to eat at night, and some who eat during the day, like me. The bottom line is that the fewer hours you eat the more weight you melt away. My eating window is determined by how much weight I want to lose and the sizes of my meals. This is why the idea of one meal a day and a tasting are so perfect for me.

The number of pounds I lose is directly related to the size of my meals and the hours I eat. The reason the number of hours you fast and eat has such a dramatic effect on your weight loss is because of how your body fuels itself. Your body has two options for fuel: glucose (sugar), from the food you recently ate, or fat that's already stored in your body. Your body will always burn sugar first. If there's so much sugar present that your body never needs to burn fat, you won't lose weight because fat-burning is what results in weight loss.

To help you understand what I'm talking about, imagine you have cash in your pocket and cash in the bank. You're not going to drive all the way to the bank to withdraw money if you have some already in your pocket. You're going to use up everything in your pocket first before you ever touch what's in the bank. That's how your body works with sugar (pocket money) and fat (money in the bank). After 18-24 hours of fasting, your body has burned up all of the sugar and starts attacking the fat. That's what you want!

There are new studies every day that continue to prove the benefits of intermittent fasting. However, the main reason it's so effective for losing weight has everything to do with **insulin**. We're not going to get too scientific here, and I encourage you to do your own research, but I want you to know that if you're someone who deals with diabetic issues, this plan can still work for you. I'm someone who, at my highest weight, was pre-diabetic, and I still have ongoing blood sugar issues. However, intermittent fasting has greatly impacted my blood sugar to the positive. If you have the same health issues I do, then you'll fit right in (of course, consult your physician before starting a new dietary plan).

I check my blood sugar on a regular basis, and I believe that's an important practice to begin. I've learned a lot about insulin and its role in regulating your body's glucose. When you eat, your blood sugar is available to either be burned as energy or stored as fat. In order to lose weight, you have to lower your insulin levels so that your body can access your stored fat effectively. The very act of eating, regardless of *what* you're eating, causes insulin to be released from your body. Fasting, on the other hand, lowers insulin, which contributes to weight loss.

Anytime insulin increases, it can inhibit fat breakdown, which is what you need for fat loss. Like I said before, anytime you eat, your insulin increases. How much it increases depends on several factors, like the food taken in and the individual person eating it, but ultimately fasting has a positive impact on fat loss.

FASTING: IT WORKS!

There are benefits to intermittent fasting that I haven't found with any other diet I've tried. First, I believe intermittent fasting is a solution for the "willpower factor." I think we all have a limit to our willpower. We can get excited about a diet for a little while, but, when we want a brownie and the diet says we can't, most times we end up failing. We move on to the next diet since the last one was "too hard" and when that one fails, we move on to another one. We blame the diets, but it's really our inability to stick with them that's the problem—but that's okay! Trying to live by a diet is unrealistic and unsustainable. Diets that restrict foods get harder the longer you do them, while intermittent fasting is the only plan that I believe gets easier with time. It doesn't put pressure on your willpower because you're still allowed to eat what you want. You're simply changing the timeframe when you eat.

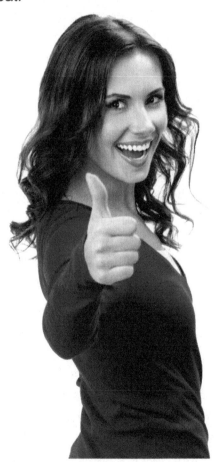

The second major benefit is that I'm finally eating less. I'm at the point where I'm eating only two meals just about every day, and they're small meals at that. See, my struggles with eating are just like my troubles with skiing. I do great while I'm in motion, but I'm atrocious at stopping. They had to stamp a big, red "X" on my ticket and threaten to kick me off the slope if I didn't stop running into people! Stopping once I start eating is just as real a challenge for me. Intermittent fasting has helped me control my eating. Now I'm even snacking less. I literally had a snacking addiction to the point where my family made up a song to tease me: it's called "All I Do is Snack" to the tune of "All I Do Is Win" by DJ Khaled (Yes, it was that bad!). Thankfully, my snacking addiction is broken now, and you won't find me snacking all day anymore.

Finally, when it comes to my health, my hormones feel regulated, my immune system is stronger, and I have more mental clarity. There are so many different cleanses out there, but I believe fasting is God's way of doing it. It's like a self-cleansing process. Don't waste your money on cleanses when you can just fast. Studies show that in addition to insulin regulation and burning of fat stores, your immune system also begins to repair itself after just 24 hours of fasting. Fasting works!

THE FED STATE VS. THE FASTED STATE

At any given time, your body is in one of two states: the **fed state** or the **fasted state**. Your body behaves very differently in both states. In the fed state, your body is actively digesting food and absorbing nutrients. How long it lasts depends on how long it takes for your body to digest food and what types of food you are digesting.

One of the factors that impact your digestion time is the kind of food you eat. Some foods digest faster than others and there's even a topic called **food combining** that explains how different foods digest better or worse when they're eaten together. I want to discuss food combining for just a minute because I did a popular food-combining diet years ago. It made me crazy! The diet centered around eliminating, separating, or combining all kinds of different foods. I learned the hard way that it made me focus too much on what I was eating instead of how much I was eating. However, it wasn't all bad because I did learn a few things about my digestion. I learned that if I eat smaller portions, my body can digest most combinations of food. If I'm ravenously hungry and need to eat a little more, protein and vegetables digest together well for me.

The other state, the fasted state, technically begins when your body has finished digesting food. However, that's hard to track. So, for the purposes of this book, we're doing a tweaked version of the fasted state. When I mention being in a fasted state, I'm simply referring to the period of time after you've closed your eating window. It's not technically accurate, but it's easier to track and it will work for the plan we're doing.

Getting to a truly fasted state is something everyone should experience. I believe that if you're constantly feeding your body and making it digest food pretty much 24/7, you're "hogging up" all of its time, so to speak. Your body never has a chance to renew itself. Fasting gives your body that opportunity and there's ongoing research to suggest intermittent fasting could help you live longer. Fasting for 24 hours, twice a week, can deliver massive weight loss while also having a positive impact on your immune system.

Pick an Eating Window and Stay in it

An eating window is a specific period of time in which all of your caloric food and beverages can be consumed. Your eating window opens as soon as you take your first bite/sip of food of the day. The eating window closes after you've taken your last bite/sip of food for the day. If that's six hours after your first meal, then that was a six-hour eating window. Let's be clear - Just because you have an eating window does not mean you should be eating two huge meals or thousands of calories because that would defeat the purpose. You can do a meal and a tasting. If I have a four-hour window, it's not like I'm just sitting here for four hours and just eating and eating for four straight hours. We still want to make sure that we're hungry, that we're eating when we when our stomach growls, not simply because there is time in our eating window. I want to make sure that I'm eating only when my body is physically hungry and not for any other reason. Thin eaters never look at the clock and say "I only eat in a 6 hour widow, it's 6:01pm and I can't eat another bite of food". Once you start obsessing you are no longer an intuitively thin person.

What you want to avoid is eating more than your body needs. No matter how long your eating window is, you can't overeat. If you eat from 12 p.m. – 6 p.m. (a six-hour window), but you consume a huge lunch, a snack in the middle, and a huge dinner then you're still eating too much. I learned quickly that if you overeat, you still won't lose weight no matter how short your window is. All of these FIRES components must work together for you to see success.

The wonderful thing about fasting is that your body learns to expect food at a certain time of day. Around 11 or 12 o'clock, my stomach growls because it's used to eating around that time. Because of this, I'm not constantly thinking about food and that's one of the major goals of *The Chantel Ray Way.* Once my eating window is closed, it's closed! At that point, I have mentally shut myself down from thinking about food and it's so peaceful! If you've never experienced this before it may sound unbelievable but trust me when I say it's a much better way to live.

I feel much more productive now that I'm not constantly thinking about food. I get so much more done and I don't even want to start eating because once I do, I know I'm going to slow down. There's a myth that you get tired if you don't eat, but the opposite happens. I'm not at all tired when I fast. I have more energy when I don't eat than when I have frequent meals all day. I think it's because the body takes so much energy to digest food. When I fast, I'm not digesting food all day long.

THE FLEXIBILITY OF THE EATING WINDOW

Different people like to do different things when it comes to the timeframe of the eating window. Some prefer to start eating in the morning and others in the afternoon. I prefer to fast in the mornings and so I get push-back from people who insist on telling me that skipping breakfast is *soooooo* bad for me. I haven't seen any negative consequences yet.

As an additional note, I do a lot of four-hour windows when I really want to jumpstart my weight loss after I've hit a plateau. If you do this, don't overdo it or you'll struggle to keep it up and be tempted to binge.

I've been asked so many times about the "perfect" eating window, and I must tell you there is no magic number of hours that every person should use for their eating window! The length of your eating window should be what works best for you with consideration of the portion sizes you eat. What is best for your own schedule, your own family life, or work routines? Maybe it's very easy for you to skip breakfast because you have long days that start in a mad early morning rush and hit your hunger level midday. So, start your eating window around 2 p.m., and stop eating by 6, 7, or 8 p.m. (depending on if you're eating in a 6-hour or 8-hour window to start). Beginners to intermittent fasting may need to start with a longer window until they get used to only eating One Meal a Day and a Tasting. Break your habits but give yourself plenty of grace while you're at it. Once you feel better, you'll love eating this way, and you can adjust accordingly.

Some people need one-on-one coaching to be held accountable, which I find is the best way to really stay on track. The second-best way to hold yourself accountable is to announce what you're doing with your eating window, and what you're putting in your body. That way, your friends and colleagues can act as accountability partners if you should graze outside of your designated eating window.

When I first started and was doing an 8-hour eating window, I did not lose weight. When I reduced it to 6 hours, I lost my initial 30 pounds, but then I got stuck and had to switch it up. Now, if I want to maintain my current weight, I have to eat in a 4-hour window and add one or two 24-hour fasts per week. For me, eating in a *4-hour window* helps me stay at my own ultimate "happy weight." Now with the 4-hour window, again, I like to tell people that they can eat what they want without depriving themselves, but at the same time they have to know what they feel. You have to find your groove and where the needle moves on your weight loss. For me, a 4-hour window is plenty of time for me to get the calories that I need while enjoying lots of nutritious, delicious food.

The 4-hour window also gives me lots of time to be able to fast, with 20 hours remaining in the day. Additionally, it is important to choose what you open your eating window with. Personally, opening up my window with a lot of carbs is going to just make me extraordinarily tired because my body has to work extra hard to process the carbohydrates after not having to digest much for the past 20 hours. A better option might be a hard-boiled egg or some nuts or an avocado, something that has some healthy fat in it. The goal is to ease your body into digestion, not jumpstart it!

Over the years, I've had to get to know my own body to understand how intermittent fasting works best for *me*, and you have to figure out what works best for you. You have to ask yourself what foods serve you and what foods do *not* serve you. I cannot eat a lot of beans and I try to stay away from all refined sugar. I did a food sensitivity test, and it said that egg whites don't work out well for me, so I will eat the egg yolk instead. But that works for *me*. What works for *you*?

The one thing that I have seen from my friends when they want to lose, say, ten pounds quickly, is to eat one meal a day and doing a 22-hour fast. They're only eating in a two-hour window. They're just eating one meal a day and they might have a little snack before that, and maybe add in a walk five days a week, or some low-key exercise like that. It's not easy, but we're talking about taking on difficult things for great end results, right? And it's only temporary to get back to a place of maintenance. As I've interviewed more and more thin women, the evidence has just continued to support the pattern of how thin women eat: they don't restrict *what* they eat but pay attention to *when* they eat. They basically eat what I call "A Meal and a Tasting." That said, of course, no one can eat only chocolate for four hours in a day and see the results they want! It's important to be reasonable and balanced. This is the formula that works best for me now. I eat two times a day: 1 medium to large meal consisting of whatever I want (depending on my hunger), and my next meal is just a tasting of about 9 bites. I might eat three bites of three different things: it's actually more of a snack than a meal.

THE BEST TIME TO EAT YOUR ONE MEAL A DAY

So, you must be asking: Do you really mean one meal a day? It is up to you to determine when is the best time to consume your food for the day. Some people prefer to eat all their daily required calories at breakfast time, some at lunch, and some at dinner. I only know one person who eats mostly breakfast and doesn't really eat lunch or dinner. There are many different viewpoints out there, and there is no absolute right answer to what is best. In my opinion, if you want to work with the body as much as possible, eating later in the day is preferred.

Our bodies spend much of the day under the control of the sympathetic branch of our nervous system. This system controls the fight or flight response and helps us respond and react to stress. During the day, our bodies are naturally a little more stressed. As the day goes on and we transition into night, the parasympathetic branch of the nervous system kicks in. This branch promotes rest and digestion. In the latter part of the day, our bodies are better suited for good digestion. I would say more than 90% of the people I know have dinner or they eat what they call "Linner". That is a late lunch with a dinner. Eating later in the day also makes it convenient to enjoy your meals with friends. You can still participate in family dinners around the dining room table, go to a dinner party, or join friends out for an evening meal.

WHAT CAN I EAT WHILE I'M FASTING?

While you're fasting, you are not to have any food whatsoever. The only things you can drink are liquids that don't have any calories. You can have black coffee, tea, water, and unflavored sparkling water. Don't have any caloric drinks like diet soda or tea with Stevia®. You also can't pop mints, chew sugared gum, take cream in your coffee, or have a hard candy. There is no sugar whatsoever allowed on your fast! Whenever you have sugar—truthfully, whenever you eat anything at all—your insulin spikes. Spiking your insulin during your fast will lock away your fat stores and that's the opposite of what you want to happen. Accessing and burning that stored fat is a primary goal of fasting. Besides, if you're constantly eating little things during your fast, you're going to counteract your ability to hear your body tell you when it's actually hungry.

It may sound obvious, but when you're fasting, you're not eating. No exceptions. Some diet books talk about "free foods"—foods that have zero calories—as exceptions to the rule. Free foods can include diet Jell-O, pickles, carrots, plain celery, and more. Intermittent fasting, however, doesn't allow for free foods. This is to truly allow your body a break from having to work to digest anything, offering it an opportunity to seek energy from what you already have in your fat and glycogen stores.

As I've interviewed thousands of women, I've learned that they aren't counting calories, they aren't counting and measuring how many ketones they have, they aren't doing a keto breathalyzer, they're not checking urine strips. They are just choosing that if they want carbs to enjoy them in moderation and focus on eating lots of vegetables and lean proteins. It is really that simple: load your plate with lots of vegetables, have a moderate serving of protein, and reduce your intake of carbs.

WHAT IS KETO FLEX?

This book is Keto(ish) but is a flexible approach to a way of eating that will keep you satisfied while you lose weight and increase energy. Finding true "Keto" friendly recipes that taste great and feel fresh can be hard (just ask anyone who is on the Keto diet or cooking for someone who is). It's a seriously restrictive eating plan that cuts out a lot of staples including some highly nutrient-dense fruits. But that doesn't mean you have to subsist on plates full of bacon alone! Additionally, there are options for healthy fruits and natural sugars. What will you eat while intermittent fasting? Crazy delicious food to the point of satiety. You will not be hungry.

One of the things that people get very confused about is the word "Keto." When you think of the word, most people associate it with a ketogenic diet, because the goal is to get the body to go into ketosis. Ketosis is a state where your body uses Ketone bodies when food or carbohydrates are low as a survival mechanism; the body will metabolize fat quickly and make ketones to save your brain so your brain can use one of two things—glucose/sugar or ketones. When you eat fewer carbs, your body eventually burns through its glycogen or sugar stores and starts using fat ketones. Your metabolism still needs the energy to power your body and brain, so it switches to burning fat for fuel. That fat comes from your body fat or fat in the food you eat. Ketosis has a ton of benefits, like more brainpower, fewer cravings, lasting energy, and weight management. You can get into ketosis in two different ways: either by intermittent fasting or by eating a ketogenic diet. People don't realize that they can get into ketosis either way!

Essentially, ketosis forces the body to use fat stores as its primary source of energy which is referred to as "fat-adaptation." Some people will say that it takes anywhere from one to three weeks to become fat-adapted, while some people can do it in a week. To accomplish this, people limit their carbohydrate consumption to under 50g per day while monitoring their protein intake. This can be overwhelming for some people, which is why I like to adopt what I call a "Keto flex" or "Keto (ish)" approach to intermittent fasting. For me, carbs and fruit are my biggest weakness, and I have had to learn how to scale back. With Keto flex, you want a healthy fat, moderate protein, low carbohydrate method of eating. Eating this way for a period of time will put your body into ketosis. 90% of what you eat consists of vegetables, protein, and healthy fat. Then the other 10% is usually made up of healthy grains, fruit, or indulgences. A Keto flex or Keto(ish) day would be somewhere between 60-80g of carbs, combined with intermittent fasting.   Here is an example of all the things you could eat to total 60g carbohydrates: a half a cup of rice (25g carbs), a half cup of diced potatoes (13g carbs), a cup of broccoli (6g carbs), a cup of cauliflower (5g carbs), and a half a cup of berries (11g carbs). Of course, this is in addition to filling up on meat and fats.

"Dirty Keto" is also called Lazy Keto, as it allows for highly processed and packaged foods. It's popular among individuals who want to achieve ketosis without spending lots of time prepping clean Keto meals. I am 100% against "Dirty Keto".

Without being consciously aware of what they are doing, the women I interviewed were eating in a Keto flex or Keto(ish) lifestyle naturally. If you asked them, they wouldn't be able to put a name to it, they'd say, "that's just what I do!" After watching them day after day, I've concluded that this is naturally how they eat. I was shocked how little and how infrequently my thin friends ate fruit. They would eat ¼ of a peach or 3 strawberries or ¼ cup of blueberries!

Go to www.chantelrayway.com, to find more details on Keto Flex/ Keto(ish) lifestyle.

As you know, I am in real estate, and one of the things that people always ask me is whether or not a rental property has a good ROI or Return on Investment. Typically, we refer to something called the "1% rule" to determine if the potential rental income can meet or exceed the monthly mortgage on a property. However, the 1% rule doesn't account for things like closing costs, repairs, maintenance, insurance, or property taxes. An easy way to calculate these costs is to multiply the cost of the property by 1%. So, if someone buys a property for $100,000 and you multiply that by 1%, then you should be able to get $1,000 a month for rent. Let's say you bought the property for $200,000; if you multiply $200,000 times 1% that's $2,000. It's often difficult to find properties that will yield a good ROI, but not impossible. Just like we look at real estate as an investment, we should look at food the same way. The type of food I eat is an investment in my body and I want to be sure I'm getting the best ROI on what I buy and consume.

As I interviewed my friends, they always asked themselves whether or not what they were eating was a good investment. Let me give you a perfect example: Let's say I was craving pizza. I could order a pizza that had regular crust with gluten and a high amount of carbs. But what if I spent the extra money on cauliflower crust? Or better yet, what if I made the pizza at home so I could be sure the ingredients were healthy and devoid of extra calories and chemicals? My investment in the pizza would be a bit higher financially and may require a bit more of my time, but the return would yield greater results than just ordering a regular pizza. For me eating, a cauliflower pizza would be just as good as eating a regular pizza because I *love* cauliflower crust pizza (as long as it's super crispy!) so why wouldn't I choose that over the more calorie indulgent choice? What is the better ROI? If the healthier option is just as good, or almost as good, why not? My friend Kim lives by this principle. "Anytime I eat chicken, I don't want it fried," she says. "For example, when I go to Chick-Fil-A, I always get the grilled chicken because I like it almost as much. The difference is so negligible that it doesn't justify eating something fried."

One of the things that I never, ever eat is artificially sweetened, fat-free, or some other fake version of real food. A quick Google search will show you that artificial sweeteners can actually make you crave sweets even more! Instead, I will use Monk Fruit or Stevia to sweeten something. Another thing that I would never eat is fake meat products such as soy or a veggie burger that wasn't homemade. These "foods" are literally filled with chemicals and are so processed that I would never touch that, even if it was fewer calories. I love to have a real, grass-fed burger once in a while, which is ultimately a much better investment due to the quality of meat.

If meat isn't your thing, you could make your own veggie burger that is juicy and totally plant-based! You can top it with caramelized onions, roasted cauliflower, broccoli, grilled zucchini, blanched asparagus, sautéed red peppers, roasted sweet potatoes – the list is endless! Now that is the kind of veggie burger I would eat! I would have to ask myself if that would be the same ROI. For some people, that veggie burger would be the same ROI while for other people it wouldn't. What is the best ROI, for *you*?

Another question I asked my thin friends is how do you decide whether you eat one meal or whether you eat a meal and a tasting for the day? They typically respond that they ask themselves a series of simple questions:

- How hungry am I today?
- If I skip a meal will I be fine or am I going to maybe overeat on the next meal because I am too hungry?
- Am I going to dinner later? Should I have a small tasting or skip lunch?

Kim is a great example of this. As a busy mother of two teenagers, she often spends her mornings getting her kids ready for school. She has coffee every day when she wakes up, a smoothie or a smoothie bowl around 11-1 pm, and later that evening she will have dinner. Almost all the women eat their "MEAL" at night and their tasting is between 12 p.m.-2 p.m. For dinner last night, she had tuna bites and a bowl of tomato basil soup. She always has some kind of protein and veggies. But Kim *loves* ice cream. "If I am going to eat ice-cream, I want to get Ben and Jerry's or Haggen Das. Something real. I am not going to eat light ice-cream. I would portion it out and maybe put 1 scoop of ice-cream in a small dish. The whole container is not a serving!"

She further elaborates on her eating habits, "If I am eating out, I always have food left on my plate. I am not part of the clean your plate club. At home, I only give myself a small portion so I might eat everything on my plate because I didn't put much on it, to begin with. Sometimes when I go out to eat, I won't even order anything. I'll pick off the plates of my family members."

Is it Worth It?

One of the things that I hear my thin friends say is that the majority of what they eat is a moderate protein, lots of veggies, and healthy fats. However, they sprinkle their day with something that is decadent. Another way to say, "Is it worth it?" is "What is the wise choice that will satisfy me?"

For my friend Kristin, she doesn't care for dessert that much and if she had her choice, she'd rather have one glass of wine and nachos as an appetizer. Kristin is *obsessed* with nachos but will not eat them if they aren't to her standards. If she takes a bite and they aren't very good, she'll order something completely different like grilled tuna bites instead. In her mind, why waste the carbs and calories if the nachos aren't amazing? Despite her love for nachos, she only has them once a week.

My friend Andrea, however, loves French fries. But she is very particular about how they should be prepared. She likes them skinny and crispy; if they are fat and wide, she won't even touch them. Because it doesn't check the box of an enjoyable indulgence, it's not worth the caloric intake. Like Kristin, though she loves French fries, she doesn't have them every day. Not because she wouldn't *love* to indulge in them, but because she knows they are an indulgence, not a regular staple of her diet.

How much is a particular food worth to you? Maybe it is worth it for you to indulge in a piece of cheesecake every now and then – go for it! But eating cheesecake every day may not be worth it once the effects of the sugar, carbs, and caloric load start to impact your waistline and overall health.

Lean meat, lots of vegetables, and healthy fats and sometimes indulging in a dessert allows you to not feel deprived while taking control of your eating. I asked my friend Andrea about how she decides what she is going to eat. The number one question she asks herself is, "how is this going to make me feel?" Personally, I like how I feel when I eat lots of cooked vegetables. But when I eat raw vegetables, I don't feel as good. Therefore, I tend to eat more cooked vegetables because of how they make me feel. When I eat a banana, I will eat a quarter of a banana. Not because I have anything against bananas, I just know that I won't feel as good if I eat the whole thing.

Thin eaters report that they hate the feeling of overeating—it makes them tired, sluggish, and uncomfortable. They regret it when they eat too much and feel it right away. They don't "diet." They just follow an eating lifestyle that feels perfectly natural to them. As you practice OMAD and a Tasting, you'll find yourself agreeing—eating too much is ridiculous.

One thing I want every reader to understand is that as long as you eat in your eating window, you can't make a mistake no matter what you eat. These days, I'll have half a donut and won't feel guilty about it one bit. Why? Because I don't eat donuts every day. The problem with dieting is people don't want to control how much they eat, so they make their food behave. They overeat on things like carrots or celery and say that because it's healthy food it "doesn't count." That's not what the Bible says at all. The Bible says to put a "knife to your throat" if you're being gluttonous (Proverbs 23:2). Period! The End! You have to practice self-control.

If I ask a thin eater, someone who is very healthy, what she ate yesterday, she may say, "A slice of pizza and half of a brownie for lunch, and half of a steak, with non-starchy vegetables, for dinner." In my head (because she's drop-dead gorgeous and super skinny) I will say to myself, "See how skinny she is, and she ate a brownie and pizza." Then I will talk myself into eating that, and I can eat it, but *only* if it's gluten-free, otherwise I'll feel awful! My body can't process gluten because of autoimmune issues. My body cannot handle it, but hers can. If I eat gluten, my joints hurt, I can't walk, my head gets inflamed with psoriasis and chunks of skin fall off, and I get massively constipated and exhausted. If you have no food allergies or sensitivities, but you avoid certain foods because you think you're being good, then you're trying to control the food instead of focusing on hunger and fullness.

You have to get in tune with your body and ask, "How hungry am I? How full am I?" This is the only way you're going to successfully lose weight with intermittent fasting. When you learn how to evaluate **true hunger**, you're going to discover you don't need to eat as much food or as many meals as you think you do. You might end up only eating one meal.

Now, don't look at it and think, "That's crazy! I might as well give up now." You're going to find out what works for you, and as you learn how to recognize true hunger, you're going to find yourself eating less and less. Start with learning not to eat more than what your body needs. To help you do that, I developed the **Hunger Scale**. The next time you think about eating food, locate your level of hunger on this Hunger Scale first.

The Hunger Scale

Never Eat Past 4 on the Hunger Scale

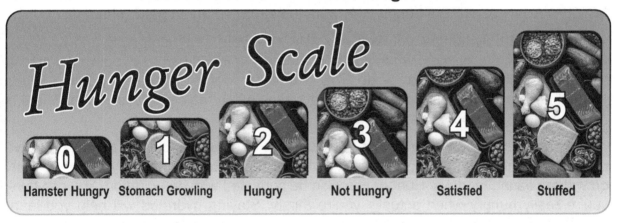

| Hamster Hungry | Stomach Growling | Hungry | Not Hungry | Satisfied | Stuffed |

0 – Hungry Hungry Hippo Hungry: Starving, ravenous, weak, grouchy. All you can think about is what to eat and how you can get it. You may get a headache, struggle to concentrate, or get "hangry" (hungry + angry).

1 – Stomach is Growling: Empty stomach. You can physically hear your stomach growling and feel an empty sensation. It's important that you feel both sensations because your stomach can growl for other non-hunger reasons like digestion. Be sure that it's growling because it's empty. Everything sounds good to eat at this point of hunger.

2 – Hungry: You're starting to think about food and certain things sound good to you. You're deciding what your body is craving.

3 – Not Hungry/Not Full: Neutral. You sense that there is some food in your

stomach and you're at peace. Your stomach feels comfortable.

4 – Satisfied/Full: Comfortably full. You might want to eat more, but you shouldn't.

5 – Stuffed: Uncomfortably full. You're getting tired because your body is using all of its energy to digest food. You may want to take a nap or need to unbuckle your belt. You feel as if you've overeaten.

IDENTIFY TRUE HUNGER

The crux of this entire book is the proper understanding of hunger. To understand hunger, you have to properly define it. **Hunger is the physical need for fuel.** It's something that comes in cycles. You're never hungry *all* the time. Hunger is also something that we often confuse with appetite. **Appetite is your mental desire for food.** You can have an appetite all the time. If you come back to work after your lunch break and someone brings in donuts, you might eat one. That's not hunger; that's appetite. Most people never know their true hunger because they don't let themselves get hungry. The goal with intermittent fasting is to let yourself get hungry. We want to be excited about getting hungry!

When you're truly hungry, you know exactly what your body is craving and what you want to eat. On the flip side, when you're not hungry, a friend can ask you what you're in the mood for and you have to decide. That opens the door to unnecessary eating. When you eat according to true hunger, you're not eating when the clock tells you to. There is no more, "It's 12 o'clock; that's lunchtime!"

It takes about a week to figure out true hunger. For some people, it's because they've never heard their stomachs growl and they've gotten so heavy that they could probably go without eating for days. Hunger can also be confused with dehydration. You can think you're really hungry when actually you're thirsty. Staying hydrated will help you learn to differentiate between those two feelings. You don't eat because the clock says it's lunchtime and everyone else is going out to eat. You wait until your stomach growls and your body is physically hungry for food. If you are not hungry, then there is no reason to eat.

Our bodies were designed with this instinctive understanding of fullness—overeating is not natural. So, you think you can change your body by eating the same way every day? It's just not going to work. You have to switch it up a bit to get the results you want. You just need some straight-up great food ideas. This is where *OMAD and a Tasting* with a little Keto-Flexing and a good understanding of the Japanese concept of "Hara Hachi bu" come in, which I'll cover later in this book.

DEFINING FULLNESS

I never really understood what the definition of full was before I began this journey. I always felt like I was hungry and could eat all day. Sometimes, I would come home from work and, if I was wearing a tight dress, I would change into pajamas so I could eat more at dinner. I don't do that anymore! Now, full is a "polite feeling" for me. Instead of eating until I'm full, I eat until I'm "barely full," or "satisfied." Stuffed and satisfied feel different. If you're eating to the point that you have to take off your belt or change into your pajamas, then that means you're eating *beyond* full.

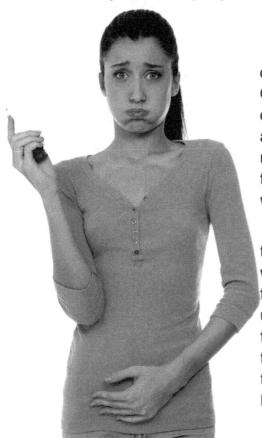

I learned my biggest lesson on fullness from one of my thin friends—my hairdresser, Danielle. One day in conversation, I discovered that she only eats one slice of pizza for lunch some days. I asked her if that really filled her up and she told me it didn't. She explained to me that when she finishes that slice, even though she's not full, she will be 20 minutes later.

Thin people don't eat to get full. I've learned that they actually hate being full. They don't like the way it feels. You have to adjust your definition of full and not expect the kind of "full feeling" you're used to. Don't be the kind of person who eats faster so she can taste more food before she's too stuffed to eat anymore. There's a real science to understanding when you're truly full and truly hungry, but it's something you'll learn intuitively.

THIN EATERS AND FULLNESS

In all of my research, I learned that "thin eaters" have certain eating characteristics that revolve around how they perceive fullness. Thin eaters wrap up their food when they're done eating and do it without arguing, pouting, or complaining. They know that they'll get hungry again eventually and they don't want to feel stuffed.

This will give your brain time to register that it's full before you clean your whole plate.

It's also important to eat slower so you can sense when your body is full. If you eat too fast, you'll blow right by "just enough" before you realize it.

There's a balance to figuring out when you're full. On days that you're only eating OMAD, you're tempted to get really, really full to compensate, but you can't do that. Even if you're someone who works out and has more muscle mass, you can't use the fact that you need more calories as an excuse to binge. It's important for you to create a habit of getting hungry. If you're feeling especially hungry when you sit down to eat, take time to calm yourself so you're not going wild on your food. Use a timer and measure how long it takes you to eat your food. Thin women take about 20-25 minutes to eat every time. Remember at around the 25 minute mark, they might take a full 5-10 minute pause and see if they are hungry, if so they eat more.

SKIP, SWAP, OR BITES
with the Cumulative Approach!

Over-eaters will:

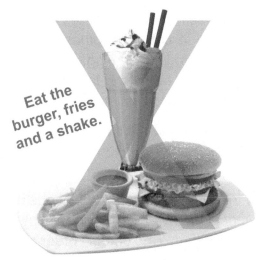

Eat the burger, fries and a shake.

Intuitively thin eaters will:

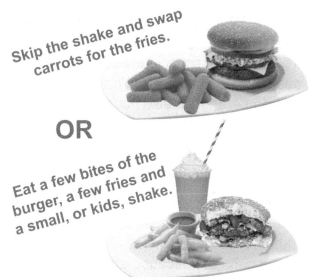

Skip the shake and swap carrots for the fries.

OR

Eat a few bites of the burger, a few fries and a small, or kids, shake.

My friend Kim says, "Rather than viewing your meal as individual components, you have to look at it collectively. I don't want to get the steak, and the potatoes, and the cocktails and the desserts. That's way too much. That's just too many calories and carbs. Within your choices, there are negotiations that have to take place. It's not a free for all! You look at the sum of the meal and then work backward. I will skip some things or have bites of something indulgent. You have to be mindful of not just the individual parts, but of the whole. If I went to Chick-Fil-A, I am not going to order the fried chicken tenders, French fries, and a milkshake and eat all of it. I would get grilled nuggets and maybe have a couple of fries. At dinner, I would either skip the cocktails or skip the dessert. I am never going to have both unless I had two bites of dessert and half of a cocktail."

For example, if I went to dinner and was craving steak (I LOVE a good steak!), I would get the steak, a vegetable (not a potato). I would eat half of the steak and half the vegetables. And then if I had a cocktail, I wouldn't get dessert. If I wanted the dessert, I wouldn't get the cocktail. The trade-offs are small but add up in the long run!

Let's say the party was buffet style and there were steak bites, cauliflower, tater-tots, mini chocolate dessert, you name it. In that case, you might have two steak bites, two tater-tots, and one chocolate covered strawberry. If everything was decadent, maybe just have a few bites of each.

But what about tastings throughout the day? Some of my tastings that are healthy would be a green spinach smoothie that is sweetened with a tiny bit of fruit. Maybe a couple of nuts or a half of an apple.

"Sometimes I will not have any fries at all, but sometimes I might eat two or three fries," says Kim. "It all depends on what I am eating for the rest of the night. So, for lunch, I might go to Chick-Fil-A and I would have a tasting. I first ask myself what kind of fries are these? These are not conscious decisions but it's how I happen to eat. It becomes so second nature that it's not conscious decisions anymore. You have to look at things cumulatively. My husband will say I am just having a few bites of cake, but he fails to take a step back and remember that he also had a few bites of this, and an entire this, and an entire that."

In addition to being mindful of how much they eat, all the women that I interviewed were also very aware of the chemicals in the foods they were eating. They would always opt for fresh fruit and vegetables, grass-fed meats, and quality condiments.

Kim might eat a few more carbs than some of my friends. If you look at what she ate in the course of a week, she eats a lot of veggies, salads, healthy protein, and healthy fats. She puts a lot of greens in her smoothies, and she likes salad. She doesn't order a salad when she goes out because she doesn't trust the salad dressings at some restaurants. She is particular about the oil she uses. She doesn't like soybean oil. She likes to have avocado oil or olive oil. If she wanted to lose weight, the number one improvement would be to cut sugar and have fewer carbs. When she thinks of sweets, she would say "I sprinkle my diet with decadent foods." One of her go-to snacks is raw almonds. She says "I'd rather not eat almonds roasted with oil. I like the raw almonds almost as much as roasted, so I'll just swap. I like the taste of oat milk; I know it's healthier so I will use oat milk instead of dairy. I swap oat milk for dairy because it's a small difference and I like it *almost* as much." The power is in the SWAP. You might think one little tweak isn't going to make a big difference, however, when you add it up, it does make a difference.

There are certain things all thin eaters won't swap. It's different for each thin eater. For example, Kim says "I will never eat light ice cream." I know what you are thinking. Why would you swap out oat milk for coffee creamer but not swap with dairy-free ice cream? Kim would say there is a difference in the taste and texture, and that difference isn't worth it. The ice cream is a splurge anyway. She says, "If I am going to splurge on ice cream, then I am going to have something I love. Also, in her mind, the full fat ice cream is healthier because a lot of times they pull out the fat and add sugar. She would rather have the fat than extra sugar. Almost all thin eaters will choose more fat than sugar. In her mind, she doesn't eat that much ice cream so let's make sure it's really good. A different example is healthy almond flour chocolate chip cookies. In her mind, that is a good swap because she is confident that it will be healthier and still tastes pretty good.

This is how she decides if she will swap or not. For example, if a regular chocolate chip cookie was a level 10 (on a scale of 1-10) to her on taste, and the healthy almond flour was (on a scale of 1-10) a 7 or higher, than she would swap it (assuming it was healthier).

If the healthy choice is only a 6 or lower, she wouldn't swap. It's not worth it. There is something very crucial you have to pay attention to on the swap. I know for me personally, if I swap something that was just OK, for something great, I will end up eating double the amount. I will give a perfect example; I bought these healthy chips one time that were low carb but tasted like cardboard. They were OK tasting, but I ended up eating double what I would have if I had just eaten regular chips. In my mind, I was thinking "well they are healthier and low carb", I ended up eating double.

Decide what delicious swaps will help you stay on track at lunch, and dinner—and during dessert time, too! Not only will you painlessly save tons of calories and see a difference on the scale, but you'll also be taking in more nutrients most of the time.

To eat the yolk or not to eat the yolk? That's the age-old question. I personally only eat the Egg yolks, only because I took a food allergy test and it said I am sensitive to egg whites, and not the yolks. The yolks contain a fat-fighting nutrient called choline, so opting for whole eggs is healthier.

My friend Kellie says when it comes to sandwiches, calories sneak in all too quickly. Next time you pack your lunch, try spreading mustard instead of mayo. Just one tablespoon of mayo can add 90 calories to your sandwich, but spicy mustard is often zero. But again, Kellie doesn't like mayo that much. So, if you think adding mayo makes your sandwich off the chart good, then add a little mayo. This is so subjective! You have to figure this out for yourself. It's a mindset and an approach that you have to customize to YOU. You have to figure it out as you go. Almost all of the thin eaters say that the second piece of bread is really unnecessary. Some of them say, I like to eat a half of a sandwich, so they will make a sandwich and give half to their husband and eat only half. Another girl will say I only eat one piece of bread by eating an open-faced sandwich. The thin eater just cut 120 calories and is happy to do it. For example, Kim says she loves an open-faced Avocado toast, but she always eats it with a fork and knife, so she will eat it more slowly, allowing her body to tell her exactly when she feels full, instead of scarfing down the whole thing.

WAIT FOR YOUR STOMACH TO BE EMPTY

When I asked the majority of people when they ate on the Hunger Scale, I would say 70% of thin eaters ate when their stomach was growling, (Level 1). But 30% said they ate at a level 2 because they didn't like to let their hunger get to a point that would make them eat too much. The key is to get your stomach to where it's completely empty. A lot of times, people who struggle with their weight have a hard time knowing when they are hungry, so the growling is a good indicator of when they are physically hungry not just mentally hungry. It's like a fuel gauge on a car. Your body will let you know when it's time to eat the same way a car does when it's on "E" for *empty*. The drop in blood sugar that occurs when you're truly hungry sends a message to your stomach to produce that empty "growling" sensation. I hear people all the time comparing their hunger to the gas tank on their car, but the better analogy is if your tank was completely full of gas and then you took your car to get more gas it would start spurting out everywhere and make a huge mess, and no logical person would do that. Why put more food in when it's already full? Sometimes people can justify putting unnecessary food in their tanks with some form of the following excuses:

- "I never eat like this." My aunt would make Iranian food, and every time she'd make it, I would always overeat. I'd justify it by saying I can't cook kabob like this or rice this good. I only eat this every couple of months, I might as well overeat.
- "It's a holiday."
- "I've been good all week."
- "Even though I'm not hungry, it's healthy."
- "I can have five slices of pizza because I'm going to the gym tonight."
- "I hate to waste this food, it's expensive."

That's the biggest thing I learned about thin eaters—they never eat before that stomach growl, unlike emotional eaters who eat for any reason at all. When you want to eat before you're truly hungry, that's the time to quote your Scriptures. You have to learn to eat when you're *physiologically* hungry (your body is hungry), and not when you're *psychologically* hungry (your emotions are hungry).

This eating plan is all about *when* you eat rather than *what* you eat. Your stomach growl is your signal to start your eating window. You'll train your body to an eating schedule as you continue to do this. If you don't get a growl when you're supposed to, then you know you ate too much at your last meal. If you're overweight and a chronic overeater, you might not have a real sense of hunger because you're running on fat and your last meal. Keep the amount of food that you're eating small so that you're hungry the next time you eat. Don't delay your eating window indefinitely if you don't hear a growl. I don't recommend you go longer than 36 hours without eating something small.

I found that there's a stigma with people about letting their stomachs growl. Stomach growling is a good thing! Getting hungry is okay! We act like being hungry is the worst thing in the world when it isn't. It's your body's natural signal to eat. Let your body get hungry, and then feed it. If you don't hear your stomach growl at least once a day then, *Houston, we have a problem!* I can't stress this enough. Your first meal of the day doesn't begin until your stomach growls. God designed your body to teach you when it needs food. The sad thing is, some people have never heard their stomachs growl because they never let themselves get hungry. Every chance they get, they're shoving food in their mouths. This can be attributed to a number of things: our immediate access to fast-food, poor eating habits taught at home, depression, anxiety, or soothing with food to avoid addressing other issues.

You can start your eating window only after your stomach growls, but you still shouldn't eat immediately. This is because you're in fat-burning mode when your stomach growls. That's your time of maximum weight loss potential and you want to prolong that for a little while. When your stomach first starts to growl, I suggest you have a cup of black coffee or unsweetened iced tea to get you at least an hour past that growl.

You're capable of bypassing your initial hunger pangs and waiting until true hunger to eat. Wait until a couple of hours after the growl, if you can. The longer you wait to eat, the further you're pressing into that fat-burning zone. You'll eventually train your body to get used to an eating schedule—mine is noon-6 p.m. or 3 p.m-8 p.m. Obviously, I don't always keep that schedule because if I go to a nice dinner, then it's usually going to be after 6 p.m. On those days, I might extend my window to an eight-hour window, or I might start my window at 3 p.m. with a light snack and be done by 8 p.m. or 9 p.m.

If you're not hearing a growl, then that more than likely means you ate too much at your last meal. It's possible to go as long as 48 hours before reaching "stomach hunger" when you come off of a binge. Most people never hear their stomach growl simply because they're constantly eating; they never actually reach an empty stomach. Keeping this in mind, you should make smaller meals so that you can reach that point of true hunger. If you eat the right amount of food, you will be hungry when it's time to eat again. It's important to create a habit of getting hungry.

There's one small thing you should avoid when you're eating: don't drink too much water. Drinking too much water while you're eating your meal can actually dilute your stomach acid and interfere with your digestion. You want everything working properly so you can sense hunger and fullness. However, outside of your eating window, you can drink as much or as little as you want. Let your body tell you when it's thirsty just like when it's hungry. When your body is hungry, eat. When it's thirsty, drink. Rocket science, right?

USE THE THREE-BITE RULE

When you cut out entire food groups and limit the number of calories you consume, you have to rely on your willpower to succeed. At some point, your willpower kind of gives up! Anytime I go the route of completely banning a particular food from my life, I go crazy, and I start losing my willpower. One day, I just explode and eat everything in sight! But when I have one or two bites of decadent foods I can say, "OK, I had it, it was fine, the end." It makes me feel like I can still have what I want.

I've discovered that the magic number for me to have the decadent foods I want is three bites. Eating three bites of dessert doesn't make my body respond negatively. This is something I can do to maintain my weight. If I'm aiming to lose weight, then I might do this once a day or even not at all. However, I never ban myself from eating any particular food. That behavior can lead to a binge somewhere down the road. Allowing myself three small bites satisfies the craving. Let's say I really wanted some chocolate mousse, but in an effort to be healthy I tell myself, "I'm just going to have this apple with almond butter instead because that's the healthier option." Sometimes, that will work, but oftentimes it really depends on how badly you want it. Because what you don't want to do is eat that apple with almond butter, say, "That just didn't do it!" and go eat the mousse anyway. Now, you've eaten the apple, almond butter, and mousse! You've eaten all those calories! It's better to just eat the mousse in a small amount rather than overeating.

In my opinion, no one ever needs an entire donut. It has way too much sugar. But doesn't everyone need a couple of bites of donut every once in a while? Absolutely! In the beginning, it takes time because you have to tell yourself that you can eat just three bites and be done. When you're starting out, you're probably going to have to throw away half of the donut to keep yourself in check.

Enjoying food is not a sin. I don't believe your attitude has to be "I can only eat to live, and I can't enjoy anything that I eat." I disagree! I think you can enjoy whatever food you want—there is nothing you can't have. You're simply learning how to eat "non-clean" foods in moderation. You don't want to have this frantic mentality that obsesses over every detail about food:

"OK, what am I going to have for lunch? I don't want a sandwich (but I do) because it has too many carbs. I don't want to have this croissant with chocolate (but I do) because it has too much sugar. I don't want a frittata (oh, yes I do!) because it has too many eggs and they have cholesterol."

Once again, if you don't have physical ailments that prevent you from having certain foods, you can eat whatever your body craves. I have tons of skinny friends who eat whatever they want all the time, but because they fast, they still maintain and lose weight.

THE THREE-BITE RULE

Here is a shortlist of things that are at about 200-400 calories that would be just satisfying enough during your eating window to carry you to that OMAD. You can open your imagination to choose those things to keep in your own house that will be right for you:

- Apple slices with 1 Tbsp peanut butter
- Apple chips (dehydrated or toasted)
- Apple and a couple of slices of cheese (choose the least processed cheese for good health)
- Warm baked pear with some cinnamon
- Rice cake with peanut butter and banana
- A banana with a handful of pumpkin seeds or nuts
- Carrot or celery sticks with guacamole, hummus, or tzatziki
- Celery sticks with peanut butter (or top with raisins like when you were a kid)
- A ramekin-full of nuts: almonds, cashews, pistachios (cracking them is a lot of fun as a distraction, too)
- A ramekin-full of a nut mix with dried fruits like raising, cranberries, elderberry, goji berries
- Flavorful crackers with a variety of seeds and grains
- Half a cup of Greek yogurt with some frozen or fresh fruit on top
- Yogurt parfait—the above with 1 Tbsp granola (see granola recipe)
- Half a cup of cottage cheese with peaches or mandarin oranges
- A stick of string cheese
- Half a cup of frozen sorbet, sherbet, or Italian ice
- A slice or two of sandwich meat, like turkey—you could add a slice or two of cheese, or on crackers
- Mozzarella cheese with roasted red peppers
- Half a sandwich with lettuce, tomato, a slice of meat
- A few slices of organic jerky—beef, venison, turkey, pork
- Some quinoa salad
- Tofu salad, or just a couple bites of firm tofu
- A small bowl of lentil soup
- A small bowl of carrot ginger soup

- A fruit and yogurt smoothie—this is one of my friend's favorites. She loves to throw in all the good things she knows she needs but might not gravitate towards in a meal like kale, probiotic powder, a raw free-range organic egg, some flax seed, or chia seed. The yogurt/fruit combination possibilities are endless (see recipes for smoothies in this book)
- A couple of hard-boiled eggs with or without a little seasoned salt, pepper, or kale flakes
- A couple of deviled eggs
- A handful of macadamia nuts with two hardboiled eggs
- A green berry smoothie
- One sushi roll with no rice with vegetables and fish or vegetables and shrimp
- Chia seed pudding and half an avocado with vegetables
- Carrots and celery with guacamole or hummus
- A spoonful of almond butter along with a handful of berries and maybe carrots and cauliflower
- A handful of Brazil nuts and a side salad with grilled vegetables

Got the idea? It's not enough for a meal, but it's just right for curbing your appetite a couple of hours before a meal. Be creative. Mix it up!

One thing that all of the women that I interviewed had in common is that if they start gaining weight, they cut back on sugar and carbs. Those two things that will add weight if you are not careful. Some people might need to decide to not eat any sugar at all except for natural fruits, which studies have shown is better for you in the long run.

One of my friends who is very thin says she'll have a couple of bites of a dessert twice a month. If it's a special occasion, she'll have one or two bites of this or that, but not having sweets every single day. Personally, once I start eating too many sweets, I can go down a slippery slope. Therefore, I don't keep them close at hand but rather stock things like nuts and fruits to curb my sweet tooth. Additionally, I don't have any artificial sweeteners at all—I just feel terrible when I have them. When I eat a meal that's high in sugar, I immediately crave a snack afterward. It's not that I'm still hungry; I just feel the need for something sweet. This is because the high-sugar meal I ate caused my blood sugar to shoot up high. So, when that blood sugar drops even just a little, I start craving something sweet to balance me out. This is a major reason to avoid eating too much-processed sugar as it ultimately leads to the consumption of more sugar, which will cause you to gain weight.

OMAD and a Tasting allows for periods of carbohydrate "fasting" and periods of carbohydrate "feasting" which is called *carb-flexing*. You will learn to carb-flex on one day after eating reduced carbs on another day. By adding complex carbohydrates back into your daily diet for short bursts of time you can feed your liver, which depends on glucose. You can still feed your food cravings—who doesn't want freshly baked whole grain bread, still warm from the oven? What about some fruit, granola, and gluten-free treats? How about polenta, kasha, quinoa, or oatmeal with milk and honey? You need to feed your diverse gut microbiome—for many of our friendly probiotic bacteria feast on the starches in grains and beans or the sugars in dairy. These carbs function as prebiotics that helps our friendly flora modify the mucosal lining of our gut and keep it healthy.

HORMONES

Hormones are such a big part of intermittent fasting and there are over 50 hormones in the body. Some of those hormones are insulin, cortisol, ghrelin, leptin. Trying to balance all of them can be overwhelming! But intermittent fasting really helps balance them out.

I was curious about how my diet affected my blood sugar, so I ordered a continuous blood glucose monitor. Even though I am not diabetic, my blood sugar has never been great, but it's been stable. Wearing a glucose monitor helps me see exactly what my blood sugar is. It's one of the best things that I've done for myself. If you are interested in learning more about how a glucose monitor could work for you, go to www.chantelrayway.com/glucose.

Keeping your insulin levels is important, especially if you're going through pre-menopause, menopause, or post-menopause. Fasting for 12 to 36 hours can help keep your insulin levels low while tapping into your fat stores for energy. By putting your body into a fasted state and pausing some eating, your hormones start communicating effectively with one another in the way that they're supposed to. It is the number one way, in my opinion, to help regulate your hormones without having to do too much. However, if you're doing too much fasting it can actually mess up the hormones and they can get out of whack.

Everything has to be balanced.

If you are in perimenopause and you're experiencing hot flashes, that is caused by an imbalance of progesterone/estrogen in your body. People say there's a laundry list of things that they experience as a result of a hormonal imbalance such as hot flashes, depression, sleeplessness, mood changes, forgetfulness, frozen shoulder (even for up to a year!). I even know people who have had surgery for a frozen shoulder. What causes this is a hormonal imbalance of progesterone and estrogen. What you need is estrogen, progesterone, cortisol, and insulin all working in balance. It's almost like a thermostat. When you have a decreased estrogen level, it causes your hypothalamus to become more sensitive. When your hypothalamus thinks it's too warm, then your body tries to cool you down.

For myself, I went to a compound pharmacy to get 0.5 milligrams of progesterone cream, and I got a compounded thyroid medication of 90 milligrams of thyroid extract and 12.5 micrograms of T3 to assist with hormone regulation. I know a lot of people who haven't taken any bioidentical supplements but have been able to achieve hormone balance from intermittent fasting alone.

Remember to look at what works for you. Just constantly play around with things and ask, "OK, how do I feel when I eat this?" It's my goal to follow the *One Meal and a Tasting* nutritional intake for the day because that is what helps me maintain my ideal weight the best.

HARA HACHI BU

One of my friends, Akimi, is Okinawan. She says Okinawa is one of the world's blue zones where people live extraordinarily long and healthy lives. I started exploring and identifying the blue zones regions of the world from some of the podcast guests I had on my show. For almost a thousand years, the Japanese of Okinawa has maintained a reputation for nurturing extreme longevity. Okinawans live a long time!

In a particular region of Okinawa in Japan, known as one of the world's blue zones because of the propensity for longevity in that area, people use a common expression, *"Hara Hachi bun me,"* (acceptably shortened to *Hara Hachi bu)*, which literally translates to "Eat until you are eight parts (out of ten) full," or "Belly 80% full." I was eating sushi one day with a friend of mine who stopped eating with just two slices of her four maki rolls left on her plate. She pushed the plate back slightly and said aloud, "Hara Hachi bu." She'd only eaten half of what was on her plate, but she knew she was done and stopped before the feeling of fullness.

Another friend of mine confessed to a similar experience when her thin daughter left a couple of rolls on her plate. My friend, having been raised as a member of the *Clean Plate Club,* reached her chopsticks across the table after her own meal was done and finished off her daughter's leftovers because she couldn't stand seeing good food go uneaten. She explained to me that as they left the restaurant, she knew almost immediately that she should not have taken that one last roll, because she did not feel comfortable—she was bloated and felt "stuffed". It would have been better in a take-out container than in her belly!

Thin eaters always leave some food on their plates. They don't finish the food on their children's or husband's plates, either. They never feel stuffed like a turkey! They eat to satiety, satisfaction, *Hara Hachi bu.*

As I explain in *Waist Away the Chantel Ray Way*, to help yourself recognize when you're satisfied and not overeat, you need to develop "stop eating" cues. It's like training a dog to go potty. I got a new puppy, Gizmo, and we had trouble potty training her at first. So, we took him to a trainer named Dorie, who told us that dogs need cues to learn to relate certain things with new behaviors. The cues can be hand signals, gestures, or sounds. For example, to make Gizmo stay, we held up a hand up and said, "Stay." To potty train a dog, Dorie told us to put a bell by the back door, and every time we took Gizmo outside to go potty, to put his nose in the bell and make it ring. This taught Gizmo that when he needed to go potty, he should ring the bell to let us know. It's the same with our bodies: we need cues to tell us to stop feeding our bodies! Since I have trouble knowing when to stop eating, I have ways to signal my body that it's time to call it quits.

How to Put Hara Hachi Bu into Practice

The biggest thing that I suggest doing is to eat slowly. I struggle with this! I eat so fast, and I say this to myself all the time, but I get a little bit better with each meal. Here are some tips that have helped me implement Hara Hachi Bu in my daily eating practices:

- <u>Eat more slowly.</u> Eating faster results in eating more. Slow down to allow your body to respond to cues, which tell us we are no longer hungry.
- <u>Focus on food.</u> Turn off the TV and the computer. If you're going to eat, just eat. You'll eat more slowly, consume less and savor the food more.
- <u>Use small plates</u>. Use little ramekins or baby bowls. Choose to eat on smaller plates and use tall, narrow glasses. You're likely to eat significantly less without even thinking about it.

When you are finished with your meal, chew a piece of gum, brush your teeth, or have a cup of coffee to deter you from eating more than you should. Coffee is a good way to end your meal, but you have to be careful because it can have a lot of sugar in it. Coffee from one of the popular coffee shops can have up to 48g of sugar! I make my after dinner coffee with cream and either a little bit of sugar, no sugar, or sugar-free flavorings or a hot cup of tea.

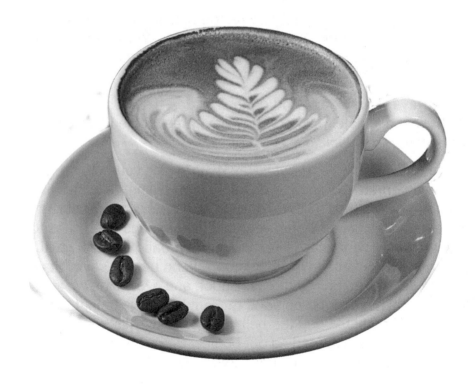

SAVOR YOUR FOOD

The best thing you can do to help you decide when to stop eating is to eat what you really want. Savoring your food is easier when you're eating what you really want to eat. I used to consider taking what I thought was an "easy route" to lose weight—taking a weight loss pill or doing a fad diet—but I realized that the true solution was to eat real food and never deprive myself. To do that, I have to savor my food.

Looking back, I'm shocked at how often I used to eat without even thinking about whether or not I was actually hungry. I ate based on how much food was on my plate. No matter how much food filled the plate, I always ate it all. I realized that the problem wasn't with the food itself. Thin eaters eat any kind of food they want and don't deprive themselves.

When you eat slower, you taste and **savor** the food. I personally LOVE chocolate mousse. Since I particularly like the whipped cream, all I do is take a little whipped cream and a little bit of the mousse and just skim the top of it. I use a fork and just take razor-thin slices. I'm savoring it. The goal is to savor your food and not deprive yourself of it. One day I was talking to my friend Catherine, who is a former Miss Virginia. We were talking about this concept, and she told me that even though she is a dentist, she loves candy, especially Skittles. She has always loved them since she was a little girl, but she doesn't just sit down and eat an entire bag of them without noticing it. She really takes her time and enjoys each and every individual Skittle! Because she takes her time and really enjoys her sweet treat, just a few Skittles is plenty to satisfy her craving!

Really enjoy the taste. See, you're not depriving yourself! Don't rip the bag open and dump the whole thing in your mouth. Take your time and enjoy it.

Thin eaters only eat what they really, really love. I interviewed tons of thin eaters and they told me that they actually **taste** and **rate** each food on their plates. The average eater tastes something she doesn't like and eats it anyway because she feels she has to "clean her plate." Imagine a plate of steak, mashed cauliflower, broccoli, and a salad. The average eater eats the foods she likes least first and saves the best for last. The thin eater eats whatever she likes the best *first* because she knows that she's going to stop eating once she gets full. If she likes the steak and mashed cauliflower, she's going to eat that instead of feeling forced to eat the broccoli and salad she doesn't want. She eats what she craves.

Usually, a salad is served before the main course of any meal and we eat it. Not necessarily because we enjoy it, but because it's there. When the main course comes out—and, be honest, that's the food you showed up for—you eat more of that to satisfy your craving and end up eating past being full. Afterward, you blame it on the meat and carbs in the main course when it's actually the salad that's the problem. You could have refused to eat that entirely and waited on what you actually wanted and eaten less overall.

Everything tastes amazing when you're really hungry! Notice that often when you take the first bite, food tastes really great; the second bite is kind of good, and the third bite isn't very good at all. Every bite after the first goes down in quality. If you were to rate taste on a scale of 1-10, the first bite is a 10, second bites are a 9, third bites an 8, and on and on. When it gets to a 7, you should be ready to stop eating. Absolutely at 6, you shouldn't be eating it anymore.

Order an appetizer. When you're eating out, ordering a small appetizer to share is a good idea. Have your appetizer 15-20 minutes before your meal arrives. Once you start eating your meal, you can eat with a lot more control because you'll already be approaching that full feeling. Many thin eaters say they order a small appetizer before dinner and share a meal.

Set a timer. Set a timer for 25 minutes, take a couple of bites, and then stop. Look up from the food and give it time to hit your bloodstream. Take the time to talk or take a bathroom break. This will give your brain time to register that it's full before you clean your whole plate.

Find a Meal Finisher and Switch Lanes. Whenever we eat at home, I feel like I don't love what I'm eating as much as if I go out to eat. This is because when you go out to a restaurant, you can have whatever you're craving. If you're craving a burger or a grilled shrimp salad, you can have those things. When you are at home, you can only have whatever you want if you have the groceries to make whatever you want. This is a perfect scenario of something that happened to me. We didn't have many groceries at home. I had enough to make a kale salad, sliced avocado, and roasted broccoli. I didn't have any protein that I wanted at the house, so once I was done eating, I wasn't fully satisfied. I just felt like I wanted something else. I ate a couple of pomegranate pieces and gluten-free coconut rice crackers, but because they tasted really good, I felt like I was starting to eat too many. Then my husband came up and said, "Chantel, stop snacking; we just finished eating lunch!" I had to find a meal finisher and switch lanes. The second I started eating too many of those coconut rice crackers, and with my husband's gentle reminder, I decided to just quickly go get one of the Pau d'Arco teas. I have a massive sweet tooth; every time I'm done eating, I always want something sweet. I have a lot of friends who have massive sugar cravings right after they finish eating, too, and the things that help with their cravings are:

- Eating more fat

- Eating more protein

- Adding cinnamon to everything

- Having decaf or regular coffee with or without cream

- Having Pau d'Arco or peppermint tea

To be true to your fast, you should only drink water, black coffee, or unsweetened tea (hot or cold). Most experts agree as for having coffee or tea during your fast — you should be just fine. Some experts say, if you drink coffee with less than 50 calories, then your body will remain in the fasted state. So, your coffee with a splash of milk or cream is just fine. Others will say absolutely not!

I also personally believe caffeine also has a stronger effect when ingested on an empty stomach, so it does a better job at helping you battle fatigue and "brain fog." This makes increased concentration another perk of intermittent fasting with coffee.

Technically, you're not fasting if you add any of these to your coffee because they all contain calories. However, fats themselves won't influence your insulin or blood sugar levels, so some experts say this is the most-recommended choice if you're looking to boost your insulin sensitivity , if you have pre-diabetes or diabetes.

While you may have heard recommendations for "bulletproof coffee"--made by adding butter, coconut oil and MCT oil to coffee--be aware that it contains over 230 calories in a 16-ounce serving (made with a tablespoon of each fat). So, you are adding tons of fat and calories.

We have to discuss coffee for a minute because the biggest problem people have with this is that they don't want to drink black coffee under any circumstances! "I have to drink coffee with cream in the morning," they tell me. "That is just a must! If I can't have coffee with cream in the morning, this diet is not for me." As I mention in Waist Away, coffee is a great way to get you through your fast. Coffee and unsweetened tea act as appetite suppressants. You should not consume any calories while you're fasting and that includes coffee with cream. Remember this is not a diet. I know plenty of people that use this approach to eating who are drinking coffee with cream in the morning. Believe it or not, you can still get results. I have an aunt who is 5'4" and 90 pounds and has her coffee this way. She drinks coffee with cream multiple times a day until about 1 p.m. However, she only has 1 or 1½ meals after that. She eats very, very little.

However, I don't recommend coffee with cream because I believe it will slow down your progress and keep you from discovering true hunger. I prefer you dig in and learn to take it black or try unsweetened tea instead. Eighty percent of the fat loss battle is controlling your hunger, and coffee is a great way to delay hunger until you're ready to eat.

Most of the women I interviewed drank unsweetened coffee with a little creamer and still stay very thin. Black coffee is what I recommend. However, like they say, "You do

ONE MEAL AND A TASTING

you boo!" Remember, you can also have green tea in the morning and maybe open your window at 12 pm and have a cup of coffee with cream. I want to say that 90% of the women that I interviewed did have a splash of cream in the coffee with no sugar because they just didn't like the taste and most of them had half-and-half organic or fresh cream. So, on the other hand, I have seen people who have taken cream out of their diet and lost that extra 10 pounds they needed to lose just from taking the cream out of the coffee. This is something you have to decide but I wanted to make clear that the people who were thin, 90% did put a splash of cream in their coffee. Remember you can train your body to have black tea or black coffee or green tea with no cream. Another option is to break your fast around noon and have coffee with cream then.

For me what I do is I have a cup or 2 of green tea in the morning, and then around 12pm I'll have a cup of coffee with a splash of cream

I have trained my body to not like sugar in my tea or coffee. I know tons of people who have trained themselves to like coffee completely black. I drink black coffee sometimes. But I rather wait until 12 pm to have a cup of coffee with cream because I like that more and that takes me to about 2pm to eat my first tasting! But as I said, I know a lot to thin women who have a splash of cream in their coffee and thrill are still super thin.

There is a timing when you should drink coffee as well. Don't drink it as soon as you wake up. You're not usually starving when you first get out of bed. Save it for later on when you feel hunger setting in, but you need to push on with your fast a little longer. That's when coffee and tea are a great help. I recommend no more than 2-3 cups of coffee a day. If you drink more than that, it won't be as effective in suppressing your appetite.

One thin friend of mine told me she is 10 pounds lighter because of the amount of tea she drinks. Anytime she thinks she wants something to eat, she just brews up another cup of tea. Having an electric teapot makes that so easy—just click a button as you walk by, set up the cup & bag, then viola, the water's ready. She drinks black, green, or herbal teas all day long. Her favorite is an organic Chai, to which she might add a little creamy oat milk. That last one would be breaking a fast, so it's best to drink it in the eating window.

If you want to learn more about what you should drink while fasting, I cover this in detail on my podcast and website at https://chantelrayway.com.

Even if you eat really well and within a tiny eating window if you sit for the majority of the day at work, your hips may widen, and you'll be defeating your attempts to maintain the weight you want. You can work out regularly during your fasting period. If you are wanting to build a lot of muscle, the best time to do so is about half an hour before you break your fast to let that exercise build muscle in what a trainer friend of mine taught me is post-exercise oxygen consumption. If you have a cup of coffee to start your morning, go work out, then about half an hour later, have a tasting. If you train at night, give yourself the same break afterward before eating—there's time for a shower, etc., anyway.

One friend of mine has always been thin, and she grew up with a thin mother who followed all of the same thin-eater concepts we've already discussed. But she has put on weight in recent years simply for not moving enough. She still eats very little, but her hips are widening due to the sedentary life of COVID shut-ins and sitting too much. Even as she was doing more baking with her kids, crafting, or whatever, she gained about ten pounds just from not running a bunch of errands for 9 months. It's the pandemic-15, like the freshman-15 we all put on in college! Well, for the New Year she decided that all she needed to change was one thing—move more! So, she reached out through Facebook to ask others to join her on a virtual walking challenge to complement her thin eating habits that were already in place. A bunch of friends signed up and started watching their collective progress together on a map of their movements. They accumulate walking points as a team and individually. That's a great way to start moving your body again if you've put on some unexpected weight like she did, helping yourself and others reach for better health! Adding in walking for about 3 miles per day is absolutely magic in helping shed pounds. Know your body. Know your own needs. Go for it!

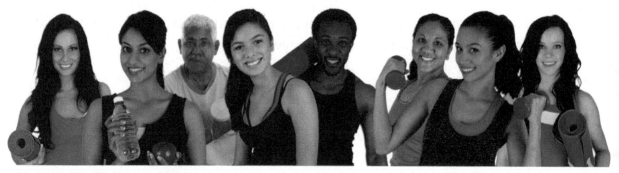

ACCOUNTABILITY

Everyone really needs a good encourager or team to help them stay motivated. I have a trainer at the gym I go to a couple of days a week, and the rest of the time I work out in a small group class. I am not good at pull-ups, and really don't like to do them, but when my trainer simply puts his hand on my back while I do them, I can do so much more. He's not really doing anything other than literally resting his hand on my back, but it makes all the difference in how many pull-ups (or how well) I can do.

This is the kind of gentle support we can all use when we're trying to make a change to our lifestyle. Your accountability supporter could be in your family even, like my friend's teenage daughter who reminds her mother that they committed together to cut the sugar back after holiday sweets binging. Your accountability team could be a group you schedule walking with a couple of times a week. You could join a fitness community to help you stick to your commitments. One friend of mine was part of her corporate downhill ski team throughout the winter when our bodies tend to go more into a slow-down. She loved the challenge and camaraderie while she kept in great shape.

Don't be shy about telling others what you're working on. Before you carpool with a friend to a party say, "Hey! Would you help me out tonight? I know there's going to be a big spread of food on the table, but I have already eaten, and I'm not hungry. I'm worried I'll eat for the wrong reasons..." And a good friend will help you out! She will give you a wink when you reach for the cookie platter but pull your hand back because you know you're not hungry.

Do you know what your mindset is? Do you know where do you get your mindset from?

A lot of your success will come from having the correct mindset. As some of you know the right thinking can either enable you or it can completely disable you. I have a friend who told me her mother stayed with her dad, who was an alcoholic for over 30 years. Her mother never worked, and her dad spent all the money on alcohol. The kids ended up having to take ketchup from Hardee's to make tomato soup, and that's what they ate. Sadly, in the mom's mind, she felt like because she had never worked that meant that she never could.

It's amazing what you won't do if you think that you can't. For example, if you said I don't think I could ever do a 24 hour fast or I don't think I could ever do a 48 hour fast, maybe you think I can't even just do a six-hour eating window. You are already setting the mindset that you can't do something, which is totally not true.

Our attitudes are moved by our mindset for better or worse. They are literally the forerunner for everything that we do or everything we don't do. I want to talk about getting your mind off the road behind you, letting go of what lies behind and saying, OK, look, it doesn't matter that I've messed up. Be committed to yourself moving forward!

Maybe you have been eaten more than you should have, or you gained weight. Put all of that in the past. Some people reading this are just stuck in a rut. The reason why you're stuck is that you've been in the same place for too long. You've gone around the same mountain and you've dug a rut and you feel like there's no way you can get out. Well, your mindset is how you view the world—it's part of your personality, social connections, upbringing, and life experiences, as well as lies we tell ourselves.

I am going to show you the DISC Personality Test.
Take a look at the chart below

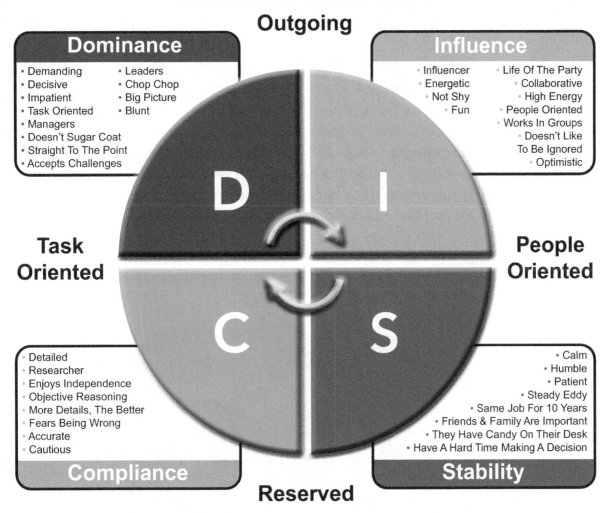

Outgoing

Dominance

- Demanding
- Decisive
- Impatient
- Task Oriented
- Managers
- Doesn't Sugar Coat
- Straight To The Point
- Accepts Challenges
- Leaders
- Chop Chop
- Big Picture
- Blunt

Influence

- Influencer
- Energetic
- Not Shy
- Fun
- Life Of The Party
- Collaborative
- High Energy
- People Oriented
- Works In Groups
- Doesn't Like To Be Ignored
- Optimistic

Task Oriented

People Oriented

Compliance

- Detailed
- Researcher
- Enjoys Independence
- Objective Reasoning
- More Details, The Better
- Fears Being Wrong
- Accurate
- Cautious

Stability

- Calm
- Humble
- Patient
- Steady Eddy
- Same Job For 10 Years
- Friends & Family Are Important
- They Have Candy On Their Desk
- Have A Hard Time Making A Decision

Reserved

For example, if you're an I personality, you tend to be a little bit happier and more jovial. That's just how God created you. But if you are a C personality, you're going to analyze the negatives a little bit more. That's just the way that your personality is. You can adapt and change that number to where you get your mindset from is the way that you were raised.

I know you've heard the saying "one bad apple spoils the bunch". I don't know how this particular phrase got its start, but it does have some basis in science. When apples or any fruit begins to decay, they actually emit gases. If the rotting fruit is mixed with a group of other fruit, the good fruit can absorb the gases and begin to rot, too.

I have this wooden bowl in my house that we put fruit in, and I watch it every day. If have one lemon that goes bad, any other fruit that's around can instantly go bad unless I throw it out. Have you ever been part of a group where one person's negative attitude affected everyone in the group? It is so true that one person's negative demeanor, attitude, or bad behavior can affect a whole group of people, influencing them to have a similar negative attitude or to engage in the same bad behavior. Like with fruit, you have to constantly pay attention to who you are hanging out with. If you are hanging out with people who constantly want to eat and think it's fun to overeat, then those people are going to bring you down. Hanging out with people who are thin or want to be healthy and don't want to overeat is important.

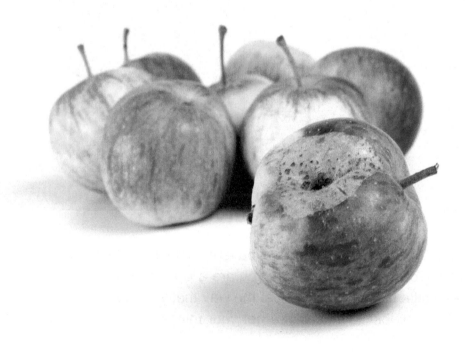

What was the mindset you were raised with? Is it the "glass half full" or "glass half empty" type of life? Maybe you were raised in a family where you often heard something repeated like, "We can't afford it." You might have asked, "Can I get this, or can I get that?" But, if you were constantly told, "We can't afford it," then what can happen when you actually do have money to afford things? You might think that even though money's not tight anymore, you can't afford it. I have a friend like that, who is very tight with money, even though he makes like $50,000 a month in passive income from rental properties. He has told me that he really wants to live on the water, but he just won't sell his house. Even though he has tons of money in the bank, he feels like he can't afford to live in a bigger house on the water. So, he has a mindset of not being able to afford it even though he can. When he grew up money was always a problem. His parents were always fighting about money and they ended up getting a divorce. He always heard his family screaming about money, screaming about mom not having the money to pay bills. He got to a point where he said, "You know, I don't ever want money to be a problem." And his work ethic matched his desire. He said he never wanted to be in a place where he was fighting about that ever again. You have to ask yourself at some point, "Do I want to think and eat like a intuitively thin person or do I want to be in bondage for the rest of my life?"

Personally, I remember going to my aunt's house—she died from breast cancer—but I remember going to her house and she had really good shampoo, great running shoes and really good products. I lived in a middle-class home, and I remember thinking, "I don't want to use Pantene shampoo anymore. Like, my hair is so much better using nicer products." I remember saying, "I want to be able to afford nicer products and I want to have expensive running shoes that won't hurt my feet and make it easier to run."

Another mindset I have had is thinking that when I'm sad, food is going to make me feel better. When I was young and I was having a bad day my mom would say, "Oh, you've had a bad day," and would take me to a frozen yogurt shop. So my mom trained me—when I was sad her first reaction was to take me for frozen yogurt or shopping. So those are some of the mindsets that I have to work on now. To say I'm having a bad day, but I don't need to go into my snack drawer and have a snack. I have to remind myself that I am only using food as physical fuel for my body now, not for comfort, or as a psychological crutch.

LIFE EXPERIENCES

What are the experiences you've gone through? These also create your mindset. For example, I had a dog named Malti that I loved very, very much. Sadly, Malti got killed in a car accident. So now when my family goes for a walk with our dog, I'm very cautious about how close she is to the road and the cars that are going by. That experience affects a mindset that I have to constantly work on. I have to tell myself to not be *overly* cautious to the point that it makes me less relaxed on our walks.

LIES WE TELL OURSELVES

Do you know that you talk to yourself more than anyone else? You need to pay attention to this self-talk in order to identify your mindset. Once you take a look at yourself and recognize where you got your mindset, you can recognize that there is some area of your life that you need to work on in order to change your mindset with God's help. Are you too pessimistic? Are you guilty of self-condemnation? When you're sitting in your car or lying in your bed, ask yourself, "What are my thoughts?" I actually say them out loud. When you say it out loud, you realize how silly some of those thoughts are and then you need to replace them with positive thoughts.

Let's imagine some of the lies we tell ourselves. One could be, "I don't have time to exercise." Is that true? We *make* time for those things that are priorities. Maybe you lie to yourself again and say, "I'll go to the gym tomorrow." The truth is, you can go *today*. You can feel better if you go. Tell yourself that, out loud.

Maybe your lie isn't that you don't have time to exercise, but instead, you'll say, "I don't have enough money to save." That's a lie. The truth is, you can always save some of what you have, even if it's just a small amount. Another lie is, "I'll give more money to God once I make more money."

The Bible says in Malachi 3, "Test me in this and see if I won't throw open the floodgates of heaven and pour out so much blessing that you will not have room enough for it."

Proverbs 3: 9-10 states, "Honor the Lord with your wealth, with the first fruits of all your crops, and then your barns will be filled to overflowing and your vats will brim over."

So, you need to offset your mindset with the opposite thoughts to fill your mind with truth. Replace those automatic and impulsive lies immediately with the truth. The world's highest performers discipline their minds, replacing negative thoughts with positive ones.

How to Get a Mindset Reset:

The first and most important thing to have to reset your mindset is *confidence*. Uncertainty breeds a lack of confidence. When you're uncertain or you have a lack of confidence, you don't make good decisions. You need to shift your mindset from playing not to lose to playing to *win*. Although that seems subtle, it's a little shift that makes a big difference in mindset.

There are things in your life that rob your confidence and there are things in your life that support your confidence. You need to identify the things in your life that cause you to feel insecure when you do them—that cause you to not make moves and not move forward. Where do you play to not lose? Flip the switch to playing to win!

Here are the things I do to build my confidence:

1. **Spend time with people who build your confidence even when you don't feel like it.**
   I know a guy who owns a large Real Estate agency and he always taunts me that I won't be able to build a company as big and as successful as his. I call him my balloon popper. Every time I talk to him, he gives me a little bit of encouragement but then also likes to pop my balloon. It's like two steps forward, one step back with him. Because of this, I'm not going to choose to spend a lot of time with him.
2. **Watch what you fill your brain with.**

I *never* watch the news. I have gone the past fifteen years without watching the news because not once in my life have I watched the news and then thought: "Well, I feel amazing!" Instead, watching the news makes me feel like, "Wow, our world is going to hell in a hand basket." Even through the pandemic of 2020, I didn't watch the news at all. This is because I don't want to fill my mind with horrible thoughts about the state of the world. It would bring me down, so I avoid it.

3. **Find things that fill your tank.**
   Identify the things in your life that chip away at your confidence and what fills your confidence tank. Know what builds you up and choose that over and over. I'll give you an example: a while back, I took a trip to Costa Rica and for the first three days, I wore no makeup and donned a slummy outfit. I looked like someone who did not care much about her appearance and I felt like I was eating a little bit more. Do you know what I realized? My confidence wasn't there. Finally, I was like, you know what? I'm not doing this anymore. I did my hair, I put my makeup on every day, I started wearing cute outfits, and I started eating healthier. My confidence was back!

   You have to figure out scenarios that work for you. I could have chosen to just slum it, but guess what? I did so much better when my confidence was back. Find things that fill *your* tank. There are things in life that, when you do them, will chip away at your confidence while there are others that will fill it up. What are the things that fill your tank? Is it being healthy? Is it working out? Is it spending time with friends? Is it spending time with family? For me, it's getting a massage or laying out in the sun that really fills my tank. So, you've got to figure out right now what can you do that fills your tank?

4. **Do things that allow you to be courageous and allow you to flex your courage muscle.**
   I get so tired of people saying, "I can't do that." I have gone on an 8-day water-only fast and people say to me, "I could never do that." Well, if you say you can't then of course you won't be able to! We must be courageous. We MUST FLEX OUR courage muscle! In order to gain confidence, you need to step out in courage.

   My husband surprised me one day by blindfolding me and driving me to jump out of a plane! Courage is jumping out of the plane when you're scared to death and having faith that the parachute opens. I was thinking I could never do that, but we were there and I did it. And, you know what? I loved it! You can do the same thing.

5. **Avoid the things that rob our confidence.**

ONE MEAL AND A TASTING

In order to do whatever it takes to build our confidence so we can take those uncomfortable actions, do the complete opposite of the things that take away your confidence. It's that simple! What are the things that make you feel good about yourself? Can you reflect on times in the past when you were scared, but you still did something scary, and it moved you forward? If so, then do it again! If not, this is your opportunity to change that.

6. **Stop hitting the easy button on everything.**

   Not everything has to be easy. Stop hitting the easy button on things that matter. I don't want to get to the end of my life and say, "Ah, I lived a good life. I had a good relationship. I was a good mom." No! I want to be *outstanding*. I'd rather try hard things and fail than hit the easy button on everything.

   Sure, there are certain things it's OK to hit the easy button on. But, for example, fasting *isn't* easy, but I can find ways to make it easier (like keeping busy).

7. **You have to get uncomfortable to get comfortable.**

   It's not about where you start, it's where you just where you finish and where you decide to go. I think there are people that are listening to that may think they don't have the advantages in life that others have. And what I'm trying to point out to those people is it's maybe a bigger advantage than you recognize. This is just the time in history when people need to talk about being uncomfortable more than anything. People think they need a particular diet when really, their mindset is the only diet they need.

   Here's uncomfortable: I go to a lot of dinners where I don't *eat* anything. Everyone around me is enjoying food, ordering appetizers and drinks, while I'm focusing on the conversation and company. Naturally, people will make comments about my lack of food and wonder why I'm not eating with them. I politely decline and explain that I'm fasting or let them know that I want what they say to be the center of my attention, not food.

I was on vacation recently and the hotel we stayed at had a great pool. We love to just lie by the pool and wait for the staff to bring out the food. However, the pool menu didn't have salad as an option. It's was the wildest thing! I don't know if it was because of COVID, but they had a significantly reduced menu. Every item that they had was like nachos, burgers, just junk foods. And so most people would say, "oh well, there's nothing else on the menu, so I guess I'll choose the least of all these evils," so to speak. But here's where you can think about your *mindset.* Do you think you cannot have a better meal just because you don't see it on the menu? What do you need at that moment? This is a service industry, and they have a full kitchen so they can serve you.

So, I asked the guy, "Do you have any salads on the menu?" He said they didn't, so I was like, "OK, well, that's fine but I still want a salad. Here's exactly what I want in my salad. I want fresh basil, fresh cilantro, mixed greens, cucumbers, hearts of palm, avocado, and grilled onions."

He went back and made me that salad. Almost all restaurants have those somewhere in the back, whether or not you see it on the menu, you can still ask for it.

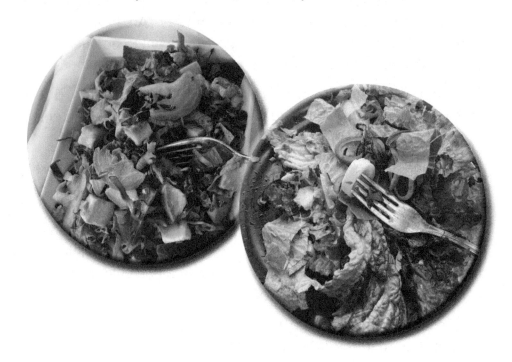

Again, it's in your mindset: Are you going to believe the lie that they can't make you a salad and just accept defeat? "OK, they can't make me a salad…" Or, are you going to push back and get them to make you a salad that you love?

The other thing is, I sometimes will develop my own drink. For example, I wanted a cup of coffee with fresh coconut cream from a living coconut. Well, the only coconut cream that they had (creamy sugary coconut syrup) was literally laden with nearly 20g sugar per serving. They did, however, have coconut waters and fresh coconuts. I had them make me my own coffee with straight coconut. I asked them to pour out the coconut water and take out the coconut from inside the coconut shell. Then I had them take all of the meat out of the coconut and brew a fresh cup of coffee, blend it in the Vitamix® Blender, and then pour it into that shell with a little bit of ice. I made my own exotic coconut coffee because that's what I wanted, and they made it for me. And so, again, it goes back to what is your mindset?

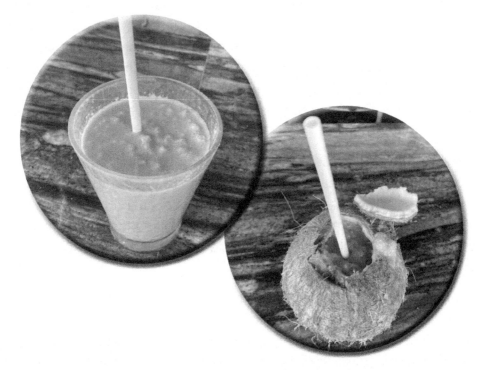

Are you just going to go, oh well I'll just have coffee with regular cream or am I going to have coffee with this laden sugar because that's all they have? No, I just keep pushing the envelope until I get what I want (Of course, I always give the people a very nice tip and they are happy as can be to accommodate).

Some of you will say, "Oh, well, I don't want to be a bother." I'm not a bother to any of these people. If you could see when I come down, they're like, "Oh, Miss Chantel! Miss Chantel, so good to see you. How are you?" They're excited to see me. Why is this? Because I've taken good care of them. They've gone out of their way to be accommodating to me, I tip well, and that, to me, is a win/win.

Let's talk about how to stop making excuses. People always come up with one excuse or another for why they can't do something, and sometimes you don't know when the appropriate time to challenge people is. How do you challenge people respectfully but still get the effect that you're after? We want people to be dialed into the idea that they can make their goals happen, but they have to get rid of excuses.

I think excuses fall into three categories: social, family and personal, and work. Let's say I am going to a birthday party and make the excuse that I have to take a few bites of cake or I have a drink when everyone else is because it's a party. No, I don't have to; that is an excuse. One time I went to an extremely expensive restaurant for a business trip that serves phenomenal food. Here I was with my grandmother, friends, and business associates all eating this amazing food family style, but I had previously decided to go on a fast. Even though it would have been really easy to "excuse" myself, I stood strong and refused to break.

An example of a family excuse would be if my husband made a fabulous dinner or my son surprised me with breakfast, and rather than sticking to my fast, I ate to avoid hurting their feelings. The fear is that I can't do that because I can't meet my obligations of being a good wife and mom. That's not true. Quality time focused on my family, not my willingness to eat every meal with them, reflects my care for them. My refusal to eat only affects me, not my time with them.

Lastly, we have work excuses. When vendors bring in the donuts and the deli trays, everyone wants to eat. I had to tell vendors to reserve these items for certain days because we couldn't have all these snacks around the office all the time. I even got rid of my own snack drawer so I would not be tempted when the stress was high. This is about accountability and a major routine change. Stop lying to yourself that you are any less engaged with friends, family, or peers simply because you are choosing not to eat when you aren't hungry or when you know the food is not good for you. People will still have a good time, they will still feel loved, and you are still amazing in whatever role you fill. You have control of whether or not you will make excuses or not, but you have to stop lying to yourself so that you'll stop making excuses altogether.

Fasting, by definition, is abstaining from food or drink for a period of time. The term "fast" in the Bible comes from the Hebrew word "tsum" literally meaning to "cover the mouth (Strong's Hebrew). In the Greek language, it's "néstis". It combines né- (meaning not) and esthió (meaning to eat) (Strong's Greek). This is the kind of fasting we will talk about in this section. We're not fasting social media or television. We're fasting in the true sense and that is to not eat.

Many different religions have some form of fasting in them. I have Hindu neighbors who fast because they feel it creates a tighter union with God. I have Buddhist friends who fast to be closer to God. My father's family is Muslim and they fast in the daylight hours during the month of Ramadan to get blessings, create self-discipline, and purify their bodies. The fasting we discuss in this section is based on Christian Biblical principles. However, if you're of a different religion, the principles still work.

I absolutely believe that you should fast with friends if you can. Fasting is not easy, so it's very important to have people around you that can encourage, strengthen, and pray with you. I believe that one of the greatest appetites human beings have is for food. It's a strong, natural desire that we deny when we fast.

I've talked to a lot of people about fasting and here are some of the reasons they told me they don't do it:

- I have really low blood sugar. It's just that my body won't allow me to not eat every couple of hours.
- I won't be able to function without food, I won't be able to go to work and be productive in my day-to-day activities.
- If I am hungry, it will actually distract me from growing closer to God because all I will be able to think about is food.
- I don't have anyone who is interested in fasting with me and I can't do it alone.
- I have a busy social life, with parties and work lunches, and people will look at me funny if I am not eating.

Most of these are logical excuses, but they are just that, excuses. Let's break them down one by one. It boils down to this- the main reason people don't fast is because it's hard! At no point do I want you to think that fasting will be easy. But nothing good in life comes easily. If you want a good marriage, it's going to require hard work. If you want a successful career, it's going to require hard work. Raising children is definitely hard. Many of you struggle with your weight and will agree that maintaining a healthy, fit body is hard. You get the point! We live in a world of shortcuts, magic pills, and secret sauces. Everyone I know who is successful at anything has had trials, struggles, naysayers, and setbacks. But they didn't give up and you shouldn't either. I've done a ton of fasting, and it still isn't easy for me! But you need to press on, hang in there, and just keep moving. Anything worthwhile is going to be hard, but worth it.

I spent 20 years in church and never heard a sermon on fasting. My first encounter with it was soon after I joined a new church, and the pastor announced a 21-day fast. It was a huge culture shock! The fast - not always 21 days - was something they did every year because the pastor believed corporate fasts were something that God honored and rewarded.

Because fasting was completely new to me, it wreaked havoc on my body. It conflicted with the thyroid medication I was on at the time and I felt miserable. Fasting is like exercise. If you've never done it before, YOU HAVE TO START SMALL! The pastor didn't do anything wrong - in fact, he gave everyone the option to do a shorter fast - but if you've never fasted before, don't try to do 21 days! It's like running 21 miles when you're not a runner. It's a recipe for disaster. Just like anything in life, preparation is key. To prepare for a fast, write down a fasting plan. Whether it's one meal a day or a 24-hour fast, if you don't write it down you will struggle to succeed. You need to write down when your fast starts and the hour it's going to end so that you don't forget. Later in this section, I am going to share some example plans to help you get started. Making a commitment is the first step to being successful with fasting. Commitment is a big problem for people in every area of life.

Transitioning into Your Fast and Sample Fasting Plans

I mentioned previously in this chapter that I dived straight into my first extended fast headfirst, and it was a disaster! To help you understand how you can build up to a long fast, I created a sample outline. Let's pretend you want to do a 5 day fast:

Week 1: Start with a 6-hour eating window for 5 days (Fasting 18 hours per day).

Week 2: Complete one 24 hour fast (I recommend fasting from dinner to dinner, or lunch to lunch, so you could start your fast after dinner on Wednesday and eat again at dinner on Thursday. Or start your fast after lunch on Friday and eat again at lunch on Saturday) .

Week 3: Do one 48 hour fast.

Week 4: Do a 3 Day Fast.

Week 5: Have a 6 Hour eating window for 5 days.

Week 6: Do one 24 hour fast.

Week 7: Do one 48 hour fast.

Week 8: Do a 5 day fast .

Feel free to try this in its entirety, to shorten it, or extend it!

The longer you fast, the more important your transition **out** of your fast is. If I just finished a three day fast, the last thing I want to do is eat a big steak and mashed potatoes as my first meal.

Your transition should be half the time of your fast.

3 Day Fast: Do a 1½ Day Transition.

4 Day Fast: Do a 2 Day Transition.

6 Day Fast: Do a 3 Day Transition.

8 Day Fast: Do a 4 Day Transition.

Be careful with processed ingredients and animal products during your transition. You just finished cleansing your body of a lot of toxins, so be careful of what you put back in. Fats and animal proteins are harder to digest. I even eat fruits and vegetables separately and pair proteins with non-starchy vegetables. Different combinations digest better than others. I don't want you to stress about food combining, but some things are common sense. Having a big ol' burger and fries and you'll feel terrible. The very first thing I try to eat after I break a long fast is a smoothie that is mostly vegetables. Then I might have some fruit or cooked vegetables. I personally stick to pretty much fruits and vegetables after a long fast.

Recently I was coming off a long fast and on the first day I was away on a business trip and I wanted to eat at two of my favorite restaurants, True Food Kitchen and the Nordstrom Café. One restaurant for lunch, and one for dinner, and both times I ordered my absolute favorite dishes, both of which had meat on them! Both dishes sounded amazing but as soon as they got to the table, I couldn't stand the smell or taste of the meat. I just couldn't eat it, and I am not sure why! I just listened to my body and stuck to the veggies. Listen to what your body is telling you that you can handle!

It's possible to experience bad breath as a result of fasting. This happens for a few possible reasons. One, your body produces less saliva when you're not eating. That saliva helps break down bacteria in your mouth. There's less saliva available to do that when you're fasting. The smell can also come from bacteria in your digestive fluids in your stomach. There are also toxins leaving your body while you fast that can contribute to the problem. Keep mouthwash handy and floss more than you normally would.

You may also develop a white film on your tongue. Use a tongue scraper or a toothbrush to clean that off. Another big side effect is headaches if you're not having any caffeine on your fast. Sometimes people forget to drink water and they get dehydrated. You could feel symptoms of low blood sugar because you're not consuming sugar and your glucose is down.

Another side effect is extreme emotions. Fasting doesn't just rid your body of toxins; it can bring up repressed emotions you've been stuffing down. You can no longer hide behind the food and those emotions rise to the surface. You may feel more emotional, "hangry," sad, or want to cry. All of these are natural and the best thing to do is pray about it, go for a long walk, or take a bath instead of running to food.

Eating food is a process of digestion, assimilation, and elimination of waste. You have four organs of elimination: your bowels, kidneys, lungs, and skin. No matter how light or healthy the food you eat is, it takes work for it to pass through your gastrointestinal tract and be eliminated from your body. That's why a water fast is so necessary. You have to give your body a break so it can have internal purification.

Even if you're a healthy eater, your food can be covered in poisons from pesticides and toxic fertilizers. If you want proof of what I'm talking about, fill up a cup with a sample of your own urine and let it sit for a while. You'll see crystals form in it. If you were to have the sample studied, they would find traces of pesticides in your urine. Fasting removes these poisons from your body. Knowing that should excite you and keep you going while you fast. You're healing your body from the inside out.

When I am fasting most of the time, I have all this energy and clarity and I am like, "This is the best day ever!" And there are other times that my staff calls "Meltdown Mode". They can see it in my eyes, I start staring in space, I am so tired, I have no energy! My staff starts laughing at me because sometimes I can't complete my thoughts or things, I say don't make sense. They will ask if I need coconut water from Whole Foods or what they can do to help! When you are extremely tired during a fast, there are several reasons:

1. **Electrolyte and mineral deficiency**

   You need to have balanced electrolytes. When your kidneys detect that you have less insulin in your body it flushes water out. You can tell when you fast that you pee a lot because it flushes you out. If you drink too much water, your electrolytes will be unbalanced. So, the first thing I will do if I am being extraordinarily strict is put some salt in my water if I am sodium deficient. I will also take these Nuun hydration capsules. They do have 15 calories and some of them have around 2g of sugar, but they have a ton of minerals and electrolytes.

   Your kidneys excrete minerals from your body to be sure you have the right balance, so you want to be sure you have the right potassium. Whenever I have my meltdowns, I know my potassium is low. When I take potassium and iron, I feel like a new person. Another tip is right before I start my fast, I like to eat foods that are high in potassium like avocados and potatoes.

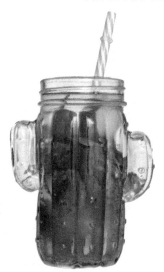

   The seven major electrolytes in your body are sodium, chloride, potassium, magnesium, calcium, phosphate, and bicarbonate. The three most important being sodium, magnesium, and potassium. So taking an electrolyte tablet when you are fasting is important because when I get in complete and utter meltdown mode and take an electrolyte tablet, it really helps me. The thing that helps me the most is 1 tablespoon of pickle juice. If I am about to quit, I take a tablespoon of pickle juice and I am like a new woman.

2. **Lack of Movement**

When you are tired and don't feel good, you just want to lay down! But that is not going to make you feel better. What will make you feel better is to go for a walk! Especially in the middle of the day when I am in meltdown mode, and going for a walk and getting Vitamin D from the sun is the best thing for me. Have you ever gone to the gym tired, and when you leave, you actually have more energy? Crazy how it works!

3. **Fuel Transition**

When you start fasting, it takes your body a while to go from burning sugar to fat. Your body has to adapt to burning fat instead of glycogen for fuel! You want your body to be using its reserved fat for fuel. When your body is in the transition from one fuel source to the other, you get really tired. Once you tap out of your sugar reserves and start using your fat for fuel, that's when you have more energy and clarity and are more alert. It's the transition time that can be rough. For me, I know that Day 2 and Day 3 of my fast are very difficult because if you think about it, your body has hundreds of thousands of calories of fat just sitting there on your body. Say you give your body 2,000 calories per day. The best analogy I can think of is from a show I saw last night where they were serving beer kegs and when one keg was emptied or tapped out, they had to switch to a new keg and serve that. So, when your sugar keg taps out, your body moves to your fat keg, but it takes a little time to switch out the kegs and transition.

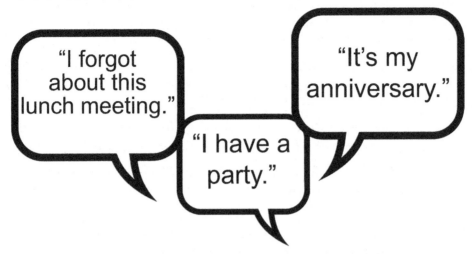

I recently went on a walk with my friend Stephanie and was talking to her about fasting. She said, "I want to do some more fasting, the main reason is to lose weight". One of the things that she was worried about is her schedule. Tomorrow, she has small group and there are always snacks and she knew people would ask why she wasn't eating them. She would have to tell them she was fasting, which could potentially be awkward. The next day she had a dinner planned with someone, the following day a lunch with someone. I told her that yesterday I went out to lunch with three friends, and we went to Aldos, one of my favorite restaurants in Virginia Beach. I didn't have anything but hot water with lemon. Later that night, I sat with my family while they ate dinner. I've gone to literally hundreds of lunches and dinners where I didn't eat, either because I wasn't physically hungry or because I was fasting. The main thing you have to do is change your mindset! I went in with the mindset that I am not eating, and it's not that big of a deal. I am going to use this time to spend time talking to my friends. I am still having fun, still enjoying myself! Instead of shoving food in my face, I get to connect and bond with people I enjoy being with. Every once in a while, I will go to another place that my girlfriends love in Virginia Beach called Stock Pot. If I am fasting, I will get a bowl of chicken noodle soup with no chicken and no noodles, and just enjoy the broth.

There's a Benjamin Franklin quote I love that says, "He that is good at making excuses is seldom good for anything else". The bottom line is you could literally make an excuse to get out of fasting anytime. If you're a busy person and you have a lot of friends, you will have a different excuse every single week on why you aren't going to fast, just like my friend Stephanie. She looked at me like a deer in headlights when I told her that I go to restaurants and don't eat!

Recently I went to New York City to meet the CEO of another real estate company that took me to dinner at Nobu. My husband took me there in Miami and without alcohol, the meal was like $400! This place is so nice, so delicious, so expensive, it's like celebrity central! This would be a perfect example of a time where I could say, "I am going to break my fast just this once since someone is taking me to a really nice dinner at Nobu." But you can make excuses, or you can make it happen. There were about six people at dinner and they were ordering tons of food and passing it around, family-style. After every dish that was passed around, everyone agreed that it was the best thing they had ever tasted. I was on the 9th day of an extended fast and was only drinking stabilizing liquids. I ordered some bone broth, and it was the nastiest bone broth I've ever tasted, so I didn't really drink it. I ended up just having hot water with lemon. I really focused on the conversation and had a great time! And it was the craziest thing, even though the food looked great, God took away my desire to eat it and it didn't even smell good to me. At the time, I was fasting to ask the Lord to heal my body, my autoimmune issues, and thyroid issues. I was also really fasting to take my business to the next level, to bring on high-level leaders, and scale our call center to go nationwide. These things are really important for me, much more important than dinner at Nobu. I had decided that the breakthroughs I would get from fasting outweighed a nice dinner out.

There is so much more I want to share with you that I just cannot put into writing. I will be going over this additional information in my new 2 Part Masterclass and brand-new video course which we will be putting new content in monthly. Once you finish the book don't forget to watch the Part 1 Masterclass that is totally free to those who purchased the book. Audio learners, there is the audio version of this book available that I narrated myself to help you revisit the chapters so you can really absorb the information.

If you are looking for more tools and resources, you can visit https://chantelrayway.com there you will find so many helpful tips and tricks to becoming the best version of you! Are you looking for accountability? Join our Facebook group to get the encouragement you need https://www.facebook.com/TheChantelRayWay

Need weekly coaching from one of our certified coaches? https://chantelrayway.com/coaching/

Below are some of my favorite recipes for you to try out. Remember you can eat anything you want; this is not a diet plan it's a way of life!

Enjoy!

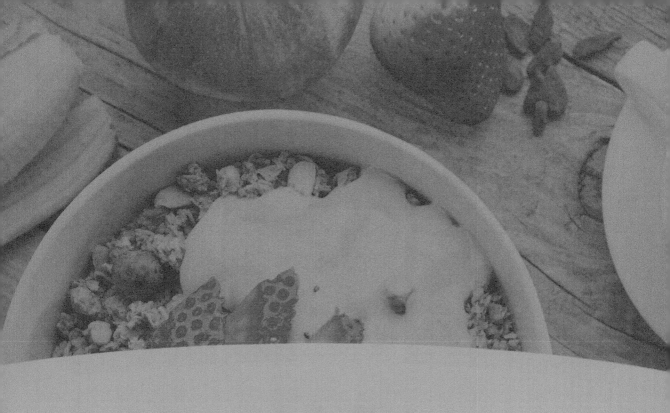
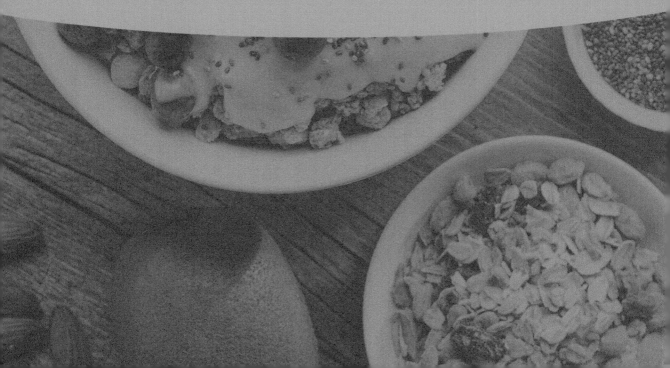

BREAKFAST RECIPES

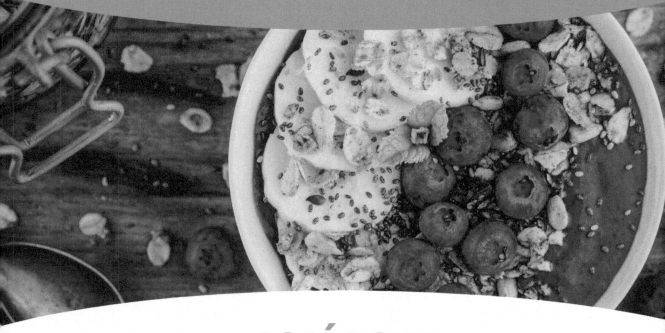

AÇAÍ BOWL

INGREDIENTS

1 unsweetened açaí frozen packet
1 banana frozen
1 scoop vanilla protein powder
1/2 C almond milk
1 tsp Spirulina
2 C spinach

Toppings: fresh fruit, granola

DIRECTIONS

Blend the ingredients above until smooth, thick and creamy.

Top with granola (see page 8),
½ sliced banana, blueberries and sliced strawberries.

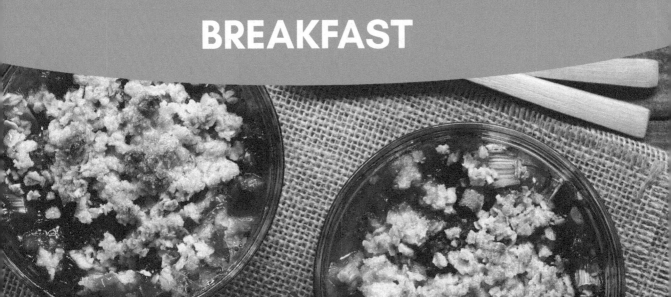

STRAWBERRY COCONUT BAKE

INGREDIENTS

2 C unsweetened coconut flakes
3/4 C chopped walnuts
1/4 C chia seeds
1cinnamon
1/4 tsp salt
3 large eggs
1 C unsweetened nut milk
1 ripe banana mashed
1/4 C coconut oil melted
2 C diced strawberries

DIRECTIONS

Preheat your oven to 350°. Grease an 8-inch square pan and set aside. In a large bowl, mix together your dry ingredients: coconut flakes, walnuts, cinnamon, baking powder and salt. In a smaller bowl, whisk together eggs and milk. Now, add in coconut oil and mashed banana. Add wet ingredients into dry and mix well. Fold in strawberries. Bake for 40-45 minutes, or until top is firm and golden. Serve warm.

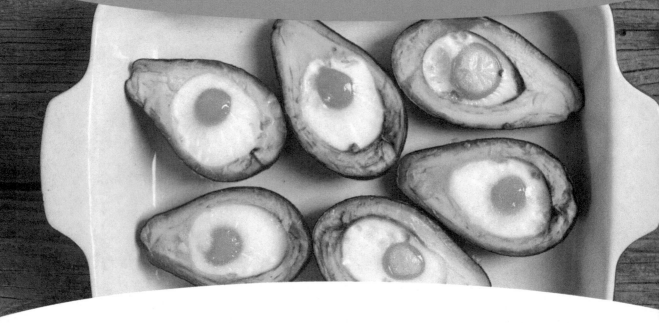

BAKED EGGS IN AVOCADO

INGREDIENTS

2 small eggs
1 avocado, halved and pitted
2 slices cooked bacon, crumbled
2 tsp chopped fresh chives
1 pinch dried parsley
Sea salt/black pepper to taste

DIRECTIONS

Preheat over to 425°. Crack the eggs into a bowl, being careful to keep the yolks intact. Arrange avocado halves in a baking dish, resting them along the edge so the avacado won't tip over. Gently spoon 1 egg yolk into the avocado hole. Continue spooning egg white into the hole until full. Repeat with remaining egg yolk, egg white, and avocado. Season each filled avocado with chives, parsley, sea salt, and pepper. Gently place the baking dish in the preheated oven and bake until eggs are cooked, about 15 minutes. Sprinkle bacon over avocado.

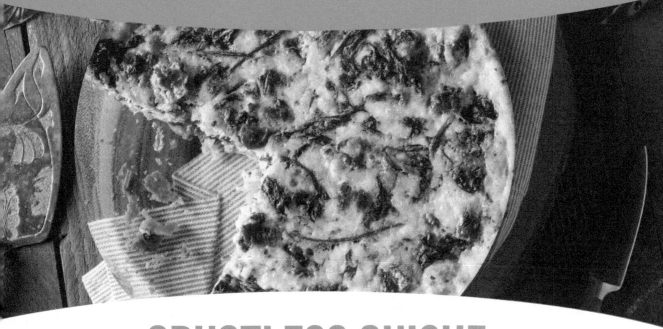

CRUSTLESS QUICHE

INGREDIENTS

10 eggs
1 C onions, chopped
1 C kale, chopped
Cooked bacon, chopped

DIRECTIONS

Preheat over to 375°. Sauté onions and kale. Whisk together eggs and combine with onions, kale and bacon. Bake for 20 minutes.

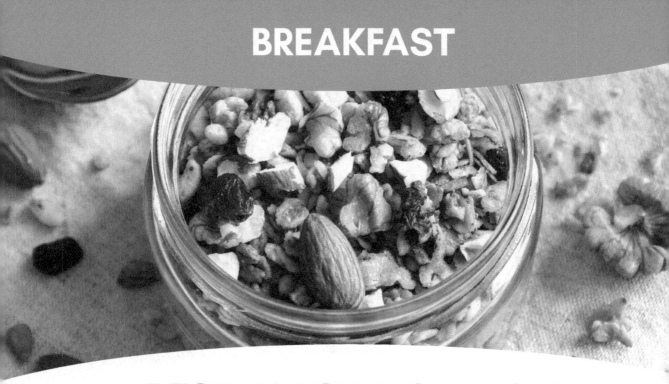

BEST-IN-TOWN GRANOLA

INGREDIENTS

1 C pecan
1 C pumpkin seed
1 C cashews
1 C almonds
3 scoop chia seeds
1/2 C hemp
1 C coconut flakes
1/2 C coconut sugar
1 tsp salt
1/2 tsp nutmeg
1/4 C coconut oil
1/4 C honey
1 tsp vanilla

DIRECTIONS

Mis all ingredients together in a large bowl. Preheat oven to 350°. Leave in oven for 15 - 20 minutes stirring every 5 minutes.

Take out and cool for 20 minutes and stir while cooling. Then return to oven 8-10 minutes stirring every 5 minutes.

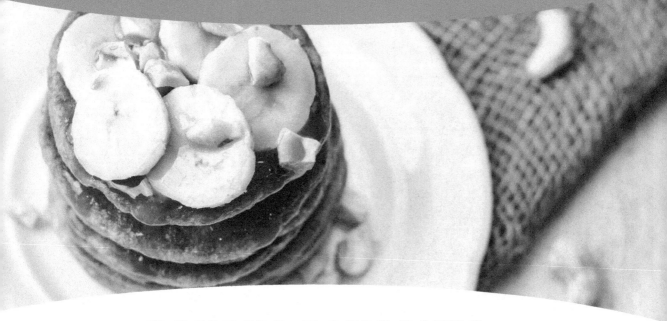

BANANA PANCAKES

INGREDIENTS

11/2 large ripe bananas
2 eggs
1/2 tsp vanilla extract
1/4 tsp ground cinnamon
1/8 tsp baking powder

DIRECTIONS

Crack the eggs in a bowl and whisk them. In another bowl, lightly mash the bananas. Add the eggs, baking powder, vanilla, and cinnamon to the mashed bananas and stir to combine. Pour about 2 Tbsp of the batter at a time onto a skillet placed over a med-low heat and cook until the bottom appears set. Flip with spatula and cook another minute. Serve immediately.

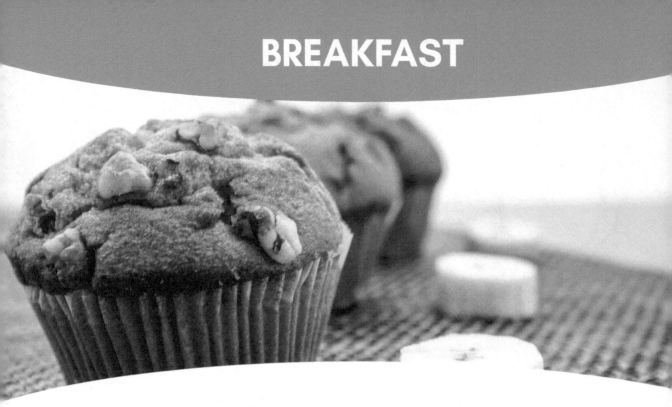

GLUTEN FREE BANANA NUT MUFFIN

INGREDIENTS

2 C almond meal
⅓ C coconut flour
½ tsp baking soda
1 tsp baking powder
½ tsp cinnamon
½ tsp sea salt
3 large very ripe bananas, mashed*
¼ C unsweetened almond milk
2 Tbsp honey
3 Eggs
1 tsp vanilla extract
½ C chopped, mixed nuts

DIRECTIONS

Preheat oven to 350°. In a large bowl combine almond meal, coconut flour, baking soda, baking powder, cinnamon and sea salt. In a separate large bowl combine bananas, almond milk, honey, eggs and vanilla extract.

Slowly add wet ingredients to dry and stir until just combined. Stir in nuts. Line a muffin tray with muffin liners or grease well and fill each C ¾ full. Bake for 25 minutes. Remove from oven and let cool for 20 minutes before removing from tray to cool completely on a rack.

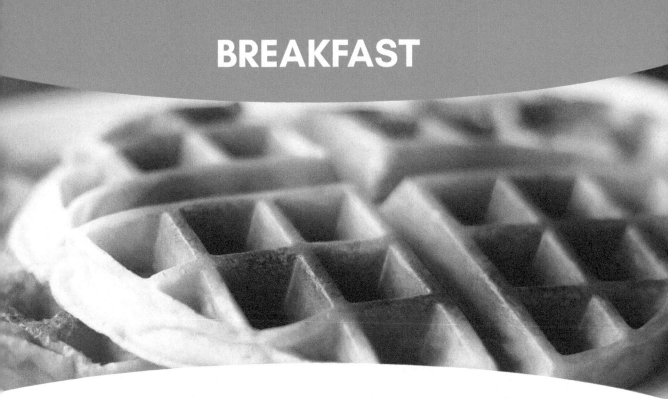

GLUTEN FREE WAFFLES

INGREDIENTS

½ C coconut milk
4 whole eggs
1 tsp vanilla extract
⅓ tsp Stevia® liquid
2 Tbsp coconut oil
½ C almond flour
½ C arrowroot flour
½ C cassava flour
1½ tsp baking powder
1 tsp sea salt
½ tsp cream of tarter
2 Tbsp gelatin (optional)

DIRECTIONS

In two separate bowls mix by hand all wet and dry ingredients separately until each is well combined. Add dry to well-blended wet ingredients slowly until all dry ingredients are just constituted into wet. Do not over mix.

Pour batter onto waffle iron and cook to your personal preference.

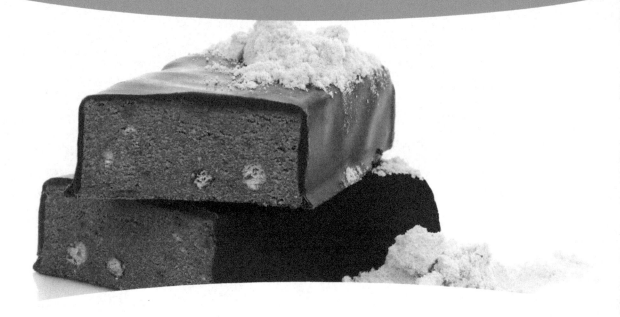

NO-BAKE PROTEIN BAR

INGREDIENTS

1 C coconut flour
4 scoops flavored protein powder
½ C dairy free-milk of choice
Vegan white chocolate chips (optional)

DIRECTIONS

Line a deep baking dish with paper and set aside. Divide half the quick oats and blend them to a flour. Combine the coconut flour and protein powder in a large mixing bowl. Slowly add milk until the batter is thick. Stir through your chocolate chips and transfer to baking dish. Press firmly. Refrigerate for 30 minutes until firm.

LUNCH RECIPES

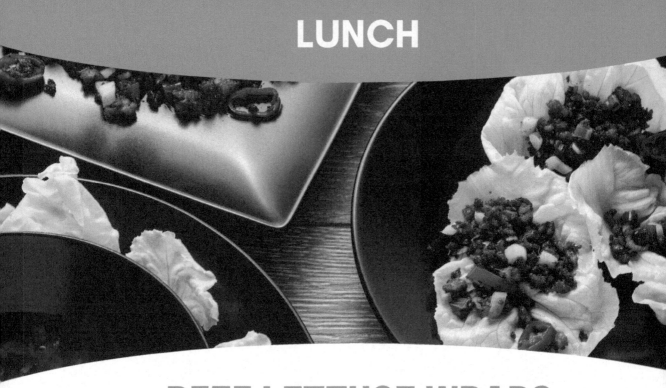

BEEF LETTUCE WRAPS

INGREDIENTS

1 lb ground beef
4 oz fresh shiitake mushrooms
1 C carrots
2 Tbsp fresh ginger
2 cloves fresh garlic
¼ C coconut aminos
1 tsp red pepper flakes
Black pepper
1 head butter lettuce

DIRECTIONS

Brown ground beef over medium heat for a few minutes.

When it starts to brown, add fresh shiitake mushrooms, carrots, ginger, garlic. Once carrots start to soften, add coconut aminos, red pepper flakes and black pepper.

Mix everything together until well-combined and cook for 5 more minutes.

Remove from heat and cool slightly.

Serve with butter lettuce. Top with your favorite toppings.

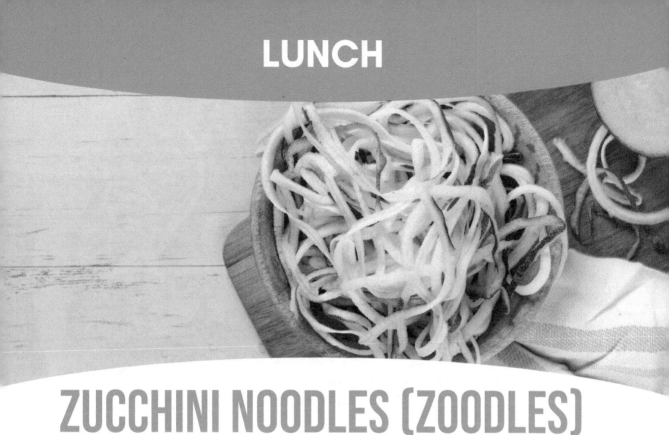

ZUCCHINI NOODLES (ZOODLES)

INGREDIENTS

2 zucchini
1 tsp kosher salt
1 Tbsp olive oil

DIRECTIONS

Cut the zucchinis into noodles using either a spiral slicer or julienne peeler. Lay them on a paper towel and sprinkle with salt. Let stand for 10 minutes. Squeeze the liquid from the noodles. Heat a skillet over medium heat and add the drained noodles to the pan.

Cook for a minute or two, until warmed. Serve with your desired sauce.

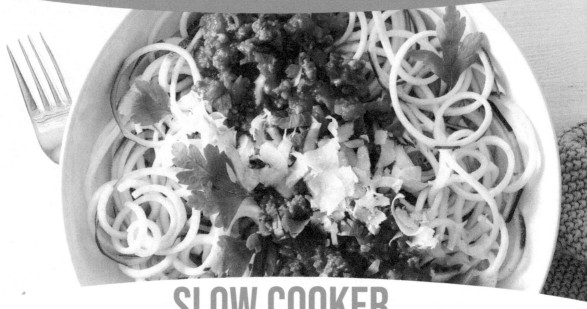

SLOW COOKER
ZOODLE SPAGHETTI SAUCE

INGREDIENTS

1 medium onion-chopped
1 lb hamburger meat
2 jars low sugar pasta sauce
3 tsp each garlic powder, onion powder,
    oregano, basil
Sea salt/ground black pepper to taste

DIRECTIONS

Cook onions and hamburger meat until
onions are soft and meat no longer pink.
Add sauce, meat mixture and spices to a
slow cooker and cook on low 4 hours. Toss
with zucchini noodles (zoodles).

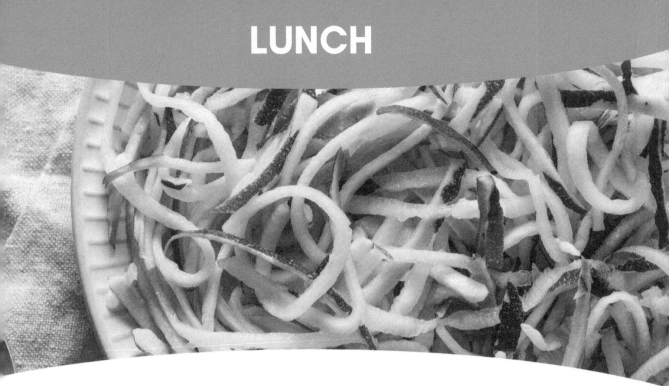

ZOODLE SALAD

INGREDIENTS

3 zucchini
¼ English cucumber, chopped
¼ very thinly sliced red onion
2 Tbsp extra-virgin olive oil
2 Tbsp fresh lemon juice
½ tsp dried oregano
Sea salt/ground black pepper to taste

DIRECTIONS

Place "zoodles" in a large bowl and top with cucumber, red onion. Whisk olive oil, lemon juice, oregano, salt and pepper together in a bowl until dressing is smooth; pour over "zoodle" mixture and toss to coat. Marinate salad in refrigerator for 10 to 15 minutes.

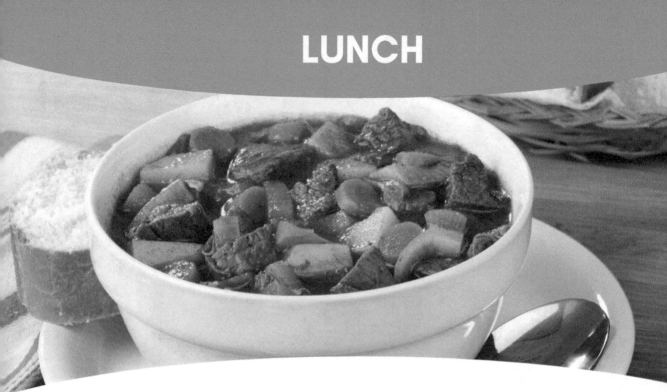

LOW CARB VEGETABLE BEEF SOUP

INGREDIENTS

4 Tbsp butter (or ghee for paleo/dairy free)

1½ lbs beef stew meat

3 oz onion, diced

2 oz carrots, diced (about 2 medium carrots)

2 garlic cloves, minced

4 C beef broth

2 Tbsp Worcestershire sauce

½ C tomato sauce

4 oz mushrooms

1 C frozen green beans

1 C frozen green peas

5 oz parsnip, diced (about half of one parsnip)

2½ tsp salt

1 tsp pepper

2 bay leaves

1½ C water

DIRECTIONS

In a stock pot melt 2 Tbsp butter over medium high heat. Brown the beef in batches, about 3 to 4 minutes. Move browned beef to a plate or bowl. Reduce heat to medium and add the other 2 Tbsp of butter. Add the onion, carrot, and garlic and sauté until translucent, about 2 to 3 minutes. Add 1 C of the beef broth and scrape up any brown bits from the bottom of the pot. Add remaining broth after the bits are removed. Add the rest of the ingredients and beef to the pot. Stir to combine. Cover with a lid. Reduce the heat to medium low and simmer 45 minutes, stirring occasionally. Season to taste.

ONE MEAL AND A TASTING

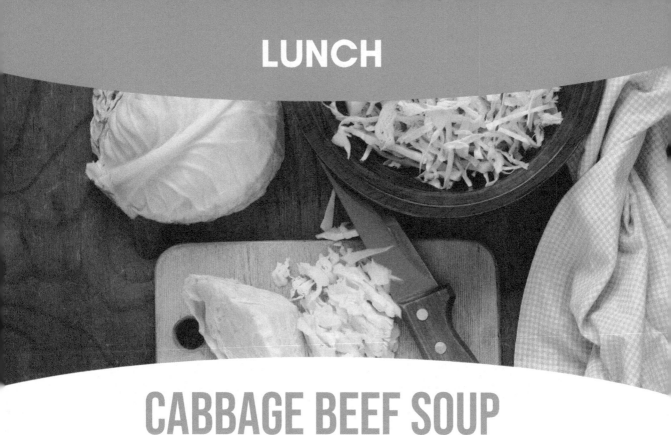

CABBAGE BEEF SOUP

INGREDIENTS

1 yellow onion
1 lb. ground beef
1 cabbage
2 cans diced tomatoes
4 C beef broth
2 Tbsp Montreal steak seasoning

DIRECTIONS

Sauté the onion with the ground beef and brown it. Then, combine all ingredients in pot and cook at least 30 minutes or until ready to eat.

All the ingredients need to cook together and flavor the soup.

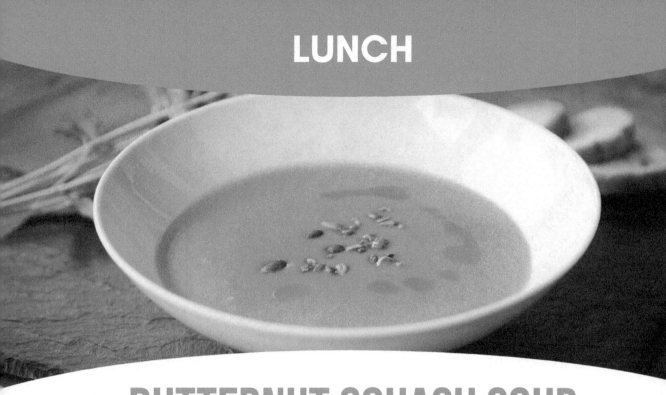

BUTTERNUT SQUASH SOUP

INGREDIENTS

3 lbs (about 1 large)
Butternut squash, peeled,
Seeded and cut into 1-inch chunks
1 C (about 4) shallots, sliced
2 tsp olive oil
½ tsp salt
3 cloves garlic, minced
1 C low-sodium chicken broth
Coconut milk
1 bay leaf

DIRECTIONS

Heat oven to 450°. Toss the squash and onion with 1 tsp oil and salt on a rimmed baking sheet. Roast in a single layer until browned and soft, about 25-30 minutes, stirring occasionally. Transfer the roasted vegetables to a large saucepan.

Add the remaining 1 tsp oil and cook over medium-low heat, stirring often, for 3-5 minutes. Add garlic and cook for another 30 seconds. Add the broth, coconut milk and bay leaf; bring to a boil. Reduce heat to medium-low, cover and simmer for 5 minutes. Remove bay leaf and transfer squash mixture to a blender. Puree until smooth.

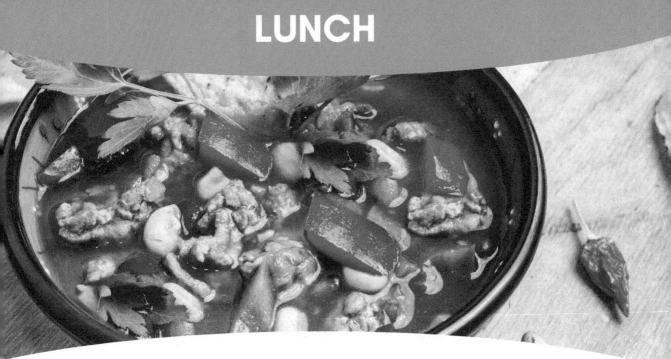

SLOW COOKER TACO SOUP

INGREDIENTS

1 lb ground beef sautéed
1 large onion, chopped
2 cans Rotel
1 can corn undrained
8 oz block of cream cheese
½ container of pub cheese
1 taco seasoning packet.

DIRECTIONS

Brown ground beef with onions and put all ingredients together in a crock pot. Add ½ to whole 8 oz block of cream cheese and half container of pub cheese. Add as much or little cheese as you like. Once cheese is warmed through, mix soup.

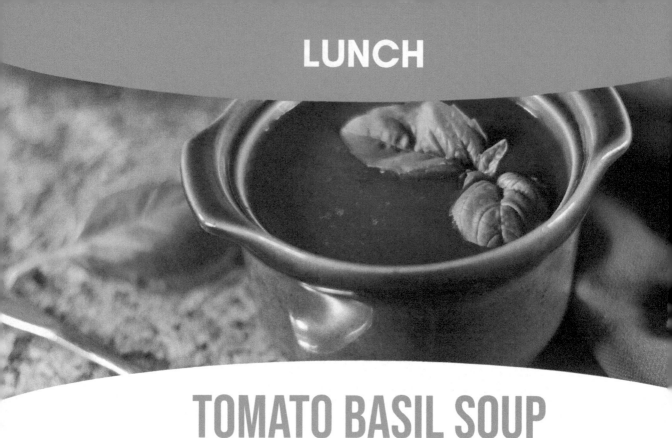

TOMATO BASIL SOUP

INGREDIENTS

6 Tbsp olive oil
4 large carrots, peeled and diced
1 large onion, sliced
1 Tbsp dried basil, crushed
3 28 oz cans whole peeled Roma tomatoes
1 quart chicken broth
1 pint almond milk or heavy cream
Sea salt/ground black pepper to taste

DIRECTIONS

In a large, heavy saucepan, heat the olive oil over medium-high. Heat until simmering. Add carrots and onion and cook until beginning to soften, 10 minutes, then add basil and cook until vegetables are completely soft, about 5 minutes more. Add tomatoes and broth, bring to a boil. Then reduce heat and simmer 20-30 minutes, or up to 45 minutes if time permits. After soup cools. Puree in a blender until smooth. Strain the pureé before returning the pot. Stir in cream little by little over low heat, until desired texture is reached. Serve warm.

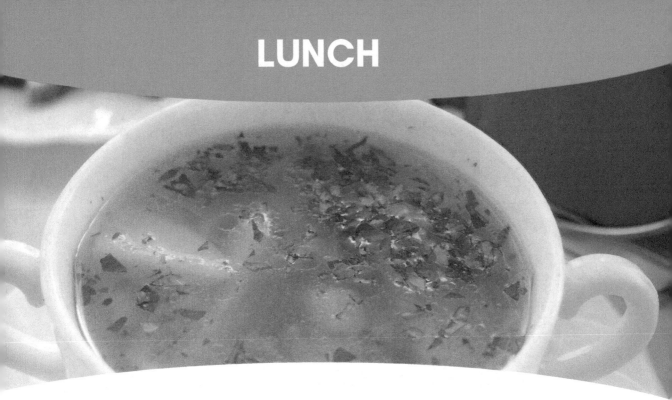

CHICKEN NO-NOODLE SOUP

INGREDIENTS

1 whole chicken

1 large yellow onion, peeled and chopped

2 large carrots, washed and chopped

2 celery stalks, chopped

½ tsp whole

Peppercorns

5 cloves garlic, peeled

2 tsp salt, divided

2 onions

Basil leaves

DIRECTIONS

Cut the chicken into 4 pieces, cutting first in half along one side of the spine and then cutting off the thighs. Place the pieces in a large pot and cover with cold water. Turn the heat to high. Add one carrot, one celery stick, the onion, peppercorns and garlic to the pot, along with one tsp of salt. Once the water boils, turn the heat to simmer and cover. Cook for 90 minutes. Remove the pieces of chicken to a cutting board and allow to cool enough to handle. Strain the liquid from the pot into a large bowl using a cheesecloth. Place the strained stock back into the pot and add the remaining tsp of salt and bring to a boil. Turn the heat down to simmer for 12-15 minutes until the carrots are tender. While the strained broth is simmering, remove the chicken skin and shred the meat. Return the shredded meat to the pot. Remove the pot from heat and add parsley. Cover and let rest for five minutes before serving.

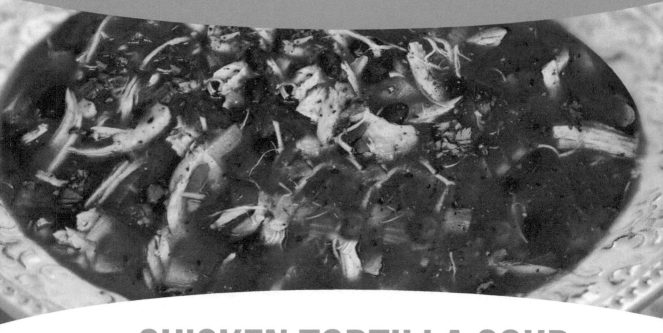

CHICKEN TORTILLA SOUP

INGREDIENTS

2 lbs chicken breast cooked and diced
1 Tbsp. Coconut oil
2 tsp Taco seasoning
1 medium onion
6 cloves garlic
2 jalapeño peppers
2 poblano peppers
2 qts (8 C) chicken stock
28 oz fire roasted tomatoes
2 limes juice of
1 C cilantro chopped
Avocado and fresh cilantro for garnish

DIRECTIONS

Mix the oil, chicken breast, and taco seasoning together in your slow cooker until well coated. Place onion, garlic, and peppers in a blender. Chop to desired consistency. Place onion mixture, chicken stock, tomatoes, cilantro, and lime juice in the slow cooker. Cook on low for 6 hours or high for 3. Serve with diced avocado.

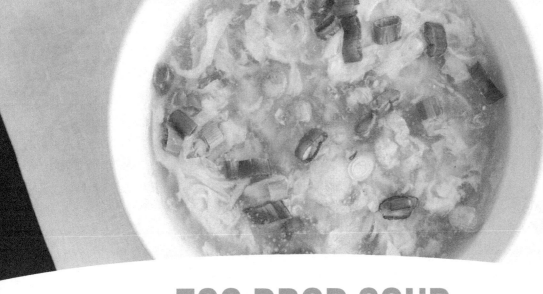

EGG DROP SOUP

INGREDIENTS

3 C chicken stock
⅛ tsp ground ginger
2 Tbsp fresh chives, chopped
¼ tsp salt
2 eggs
1 egg yolk

DIRECTIONS

Pour the chicken stock into a large saucepan over a medium-high heat. Add the ginger, chives and salt to the liquid and allow it to come to a boil. In a small bowl, whisk together the eggs and yolk. As the broth continues to boil, use a fork and drizzle the eggs into the pot. The eggs should cook immediately.

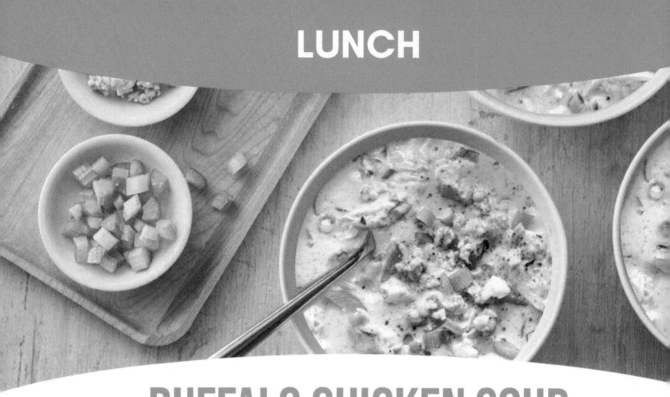

BUFFALO CHICKEN SOUP

INGREDIENTS

2 Tbsp ghee
1 C diced carrots
1 C diced celery
½ white onion, minced
3 garlic cloves, minced
4 C cauliflower florets
32 oz chicken bone broth
⅔ C frank's red hot sauce
Salt and pepper, to taste
1 roasted chicken, pulled & shredded

For garnish:
Fresh cilantro
Chopped green onions
Hot pepper sauce
Avocado oil ranch

DIRECTIONS

Place ghee in the basin of the Instant Pot® then press the sauté button. Once the ghee begins to melt, add the carrots, celery, onion and garlic and sauté for about 5 minutes, until onion becomes translucent. Press the keep warm/cancel button, add the cauliflower, chicken broth, hot sauce and a hefty pinch of both salt and pepper, then secure the lid, close off the pressure valve and press the soup button. This will cook for 30 minutes once it comes up to pressure. Once the soup is done cooking, you can let it naturally release or do a quick release. Once you remove the lid, use an immersion blender to blend the soup until completely smooth. Taste to see if the soup needs any extra salt or pepper. Turn the soup back onto the sauté function, add the rotisserie chicken and let cook down for 8-10 minutes, stirring every 2 minutes to keep from sticking. Press the keep warm/cancel button before serving. Garnish soup with a swirl of ranch, hot sauce, green onions and cilantro.

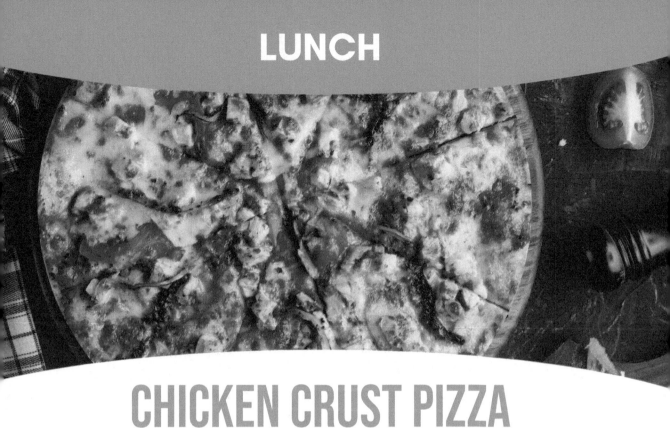

CHICKEN CRUST PIZZA

INGREDIENTS

10 oz canned chicken
1 oz grated Parmesan
1 large egg
Top with your favorite toppings like fresh
   mozzarella, tomato and basil.

DIRECTIONS

Preheat over to 350° . Thoroughly drain the canned chicken, getting as much moisture out as possible. Spread chicken on a baking sheet lined with a silicon mat. Bake for 10 minutes to dry out the chicken. Remove chicken and place in a mixing bowl. Increase heat of oven to 500°. Add cheese and egg to the bowl and mix. Pour mixture onto baking sheet lined with a silicon mat and spread thin. Placing parchment paper on top and using a rolling pin makes this easier. Optional: with a spatula press the edges of the crust in to for a ridge for the crust. This is beneficial if you're using toppings that may slide off (e.g. eggs). Bake the crust for 8-10 minutes at 500°. Remove crust from oven. Add desired toppings and bake for another 6-10 minutes at 500° G. Toppings will dictate final cook time. Remove from oven and allow to cool for a few minutes.

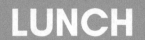

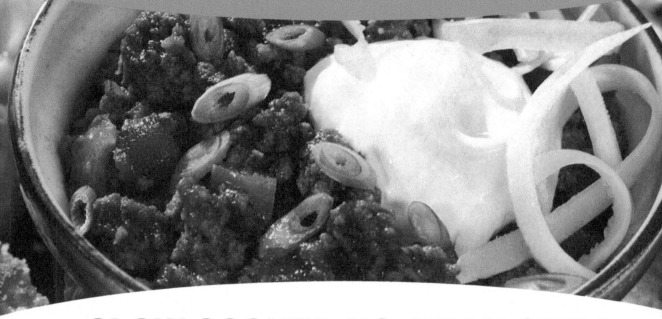

SLOW COOKER NO-BEAN CHILI

INGREDIENTS

2½ lbs ground beef
1 medium red onion, chopped and divided
4 Tbsp minced garlic
3 large ribs of celery, diced
¼ C pickled jalapeno slices
6 oz can tomato paste
14½ oz can tomatoes and green chilies
14½ oz can stewed tomatoes with Mexican seasoning
2 Tbsp Worcestershire sauce or coconut aminos
4 Tbsp chili powder
2 Tbsp cumin, mounded
2 tsp sea salt
½ tsp cayenne
1 tsp garlic powder
1 tsp onion powder
1 tsp oregano
1 tsp black pepper

DIRECTIONS

Heat slow cooker on low setting. In a large skillet over medium-high heat, add ground beef, half of the onions, 2 Tbsp Minced garlic, and salt and pepper. Once the beef is browned, drain excess grease from pan. Transfer ground beef mixture to slow cooker. Add remaining onions, garlic, celery, jalapenos, tomato paste, tomatoes and chilies (with liquid), stewed tomatoes (with liquid), Worcestershire sauce, chili powder, cumin, salt, cayenne, garlic powder, onion powder, oregano, and black pepper. Stir until all ingredients are well combined. Cook on low 6-8 hours.

ONE MEAL AND A TASTING

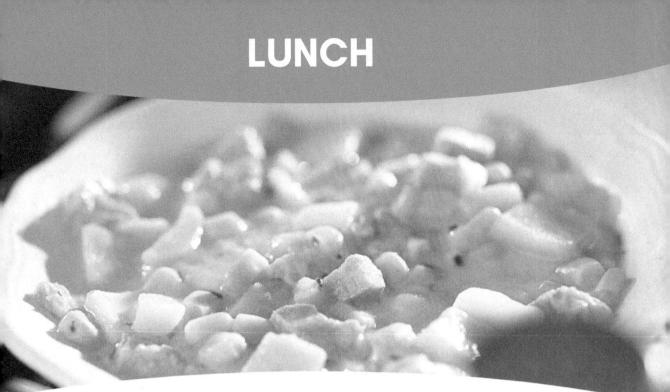

CAULIFLOWER AND CORN CHOWDER

INGREDIENTS

2 heads of cauliflower, chopped
½ can of corn (drained)
4 C chicken broth
Sea salt/ground black pepper to taste
8 oz cream cheese
Cheddar cheese optional

DIRECTIONS

Combine cauliflower, corn, broth, and salt/pepper in pot and cook until cauliflower is soft. Then take off stove and stir in cream cheese until melted. You can garnish in bowls with cheddar cheese.

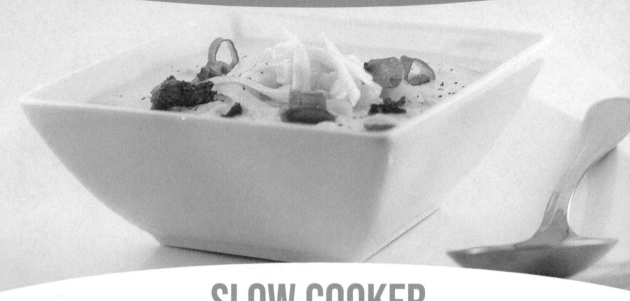

SLOW COOKER VEGETABLE CHOWDER

INGREDIENTS

2 Tbsp olive oil
1 medium yellow onion, diced (about 2 C)
1 Medium red bell pepper, seeded and diced
3 C of chopped cauliflower
4 C of broccoli, chopped
4 C vegetable broth
1 tsp ground cumin
1/2 tsp smoked paprika
1/8 tsp cayenne pepper
1 tsp kosher salt
1 C almond milk
Sea salt/ground black pepper to taste
Chopped red bell pepper to garnish
Corn kernels to garnish
Sliced scallions to garnish

DIRECTIONS

Heat the olive oil in a medium sauté pan over medium heat. Add the onion and cook, stirring occasionally, until translucent and soft, about 5 minutes. Transfer the onion to the slow cooker, along with the red bell pepper, cauliflower, 1 C broccoli, broth, cumin, smoked paprika, cayenne pepper, and salt. Cook on low for 8-10 hours or on high for 4-6 hours, until the cauliflower is tender. Turn the slow cooker off and remove the lid. Allow the soup to cool slightly. Using an immersion blender or working in batches with a regular blender, pureé the soup. Return it to the slow cooker and turn it back on. Stir in the remaining 3 C broccoli and almond milk. Cover the slow cooker and cook on low for another 20-30 minutes, until heated through. Season with salt and pepper to taste. Serve topped with additional broccoli, diced bell pepper, and/or sliced scallions.

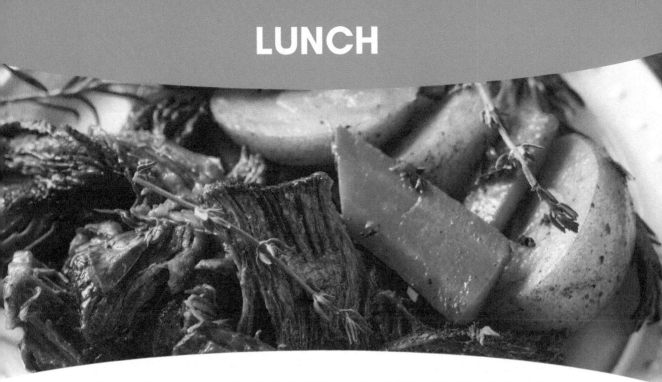

SLOW COOKER POT ROAST

INGREDIENTS

1 chuck roast or pot roast
1 package onion soup mix
1 green bell pepper, chopped
1 carrot, chopped
Pepper
Water

DIRECTIONS

Place all ingredients in slow cooker and cover with water ¾ way up the meat. Place lid on and cook on low for 8-10 hours. When finished, remove meat and slice. It will usually fall apart. Pour the liquid and veggies in a blender and pureé. May need to add water if it tastes too concentrated, and then thicken with corn starch if too thin.

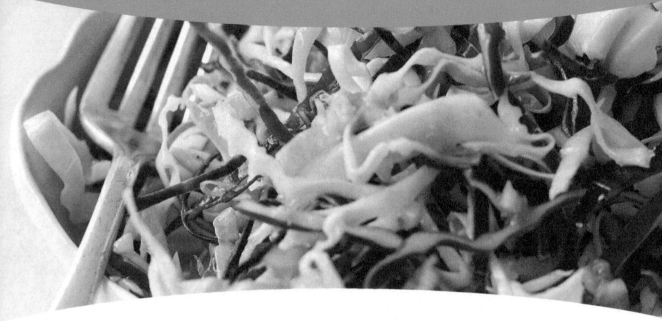

CABBAGE CRUNCH

INGREDIENTS

8 C green cabbage, shredded
   (½ a large head)
1 tsp black sesame seed, toasted
4 scallions, sliced with some green stems
¼ C sliced almonds

Honey Dressing
¼ C olive oil
1 Tbsp sesame oil
2 Tbsp apple cider vinegar
1 Tbsp honey
Sea salt, to taste

DIRECTIONS

Toss all salad ingredients together with dressing. Keep refrigerated until ready to serve.

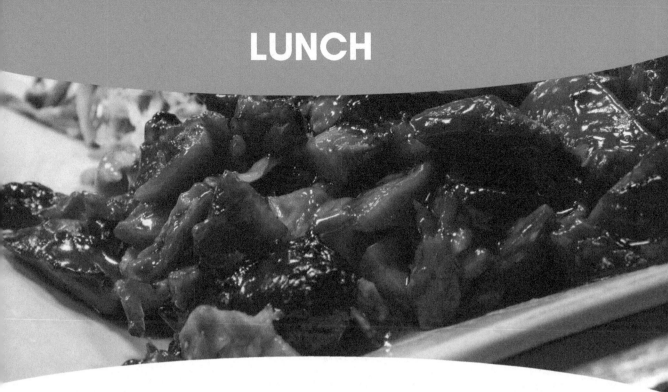

TERIYAKI CHICKEN KABOBS

INGREDIENTS

Boneless skinless chicken breasts
Green peppers
Onion
Fresh pineapple
Jasmine or basmati rice

Teriyaki-style sauce
½ C coconut aminos
2 Tbsp white wine vinegar
Juice of 1 lemon
¼ C fresh pineapple juice
¾ tsp. Ground ginger

DIRECTIONS

Cut boneless skinless breasts into chunks and pour ½ of teriyaki-style sauce into resealable baggies and marinate over night. Take green peppers, onion and fresh pineapple and cut into chucks and put on skewers with chicken. Grill all then pour leftover sauce over top. Serve with rice.

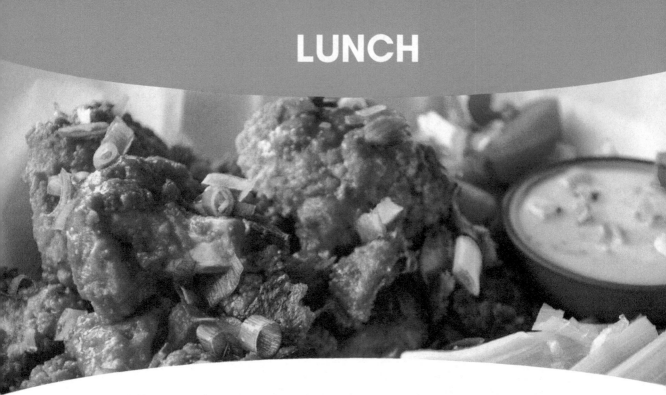

CAULIFLOWER BUFFALO WINGS

INGREDIENTS

1 large head of cauliflower, chopped into florets
1 C almond milk
¾ C Rice flour
1 tsp onion powder
1 tsp garlic powder
½ tsp salt
¼ tsp paprika
⅛ tsp ground black pepper

For the Buffalo wings sauce:
½ C water
¼ C apple cider vinegar
¼ C tomato paste
2 Tbsp tamari
2 Tbsp tahini
2 tsp paprika
3 tsp garlic powder

DIRECTIONS

Preheat the oven to 450°. Mix the batter ingredients in a bowl until well combined. Dip each floret into the batter and coat evenly. Shake off excess and place on a parchment-lined baking sheet. Bake for 20 minutes, flipping the florets over halfway through.

To make the Buffalo wings sauce you can add the ingredients to a blender and blend until smooth. Toss the baked florets in the sauce,. Shake off excess and place back on the baking sheet.

Bake for another 20 minutes or until golden brown flipping the florets over halfway through and make sure they are crispy.

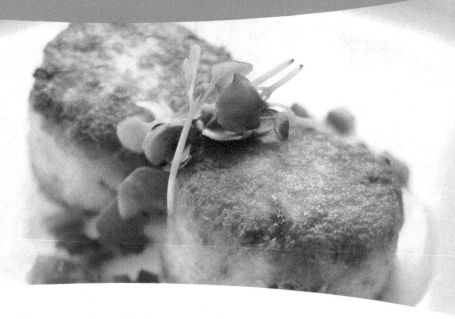

CRAB CAKES

INGREDIENTS

¼ C celery, finely diced
¼ C onion, finely diced
1 large egg, lightly beaten
2 Tbsp mayonnaise, preferably homemade
2 Tbsp coconut milk
6 oz lump crab meat
1 tsp Old Bay® seasoning
2 tsp dill pickle, finely chopped
2 Tbsp fresh parsley, finely chopped
2 Tbsp coconut flour
½ tsp kosher salt
Few grinds black pepper
2 Tbsp coconut oil

DIRECTIONS

Gently combine all of the ingredients except the coconut oil in a medium mixing bowl. Carefully shape into three patties; cover with plastic wrap and refrigerate for 30 minutes. Heat the coconut oil in a large, heavy skillet over medium-high heat. Fry the crab cakes until golden brown, about 4 minutes per side.

Serve with fresh lemon and tartar or cocktail sauce.

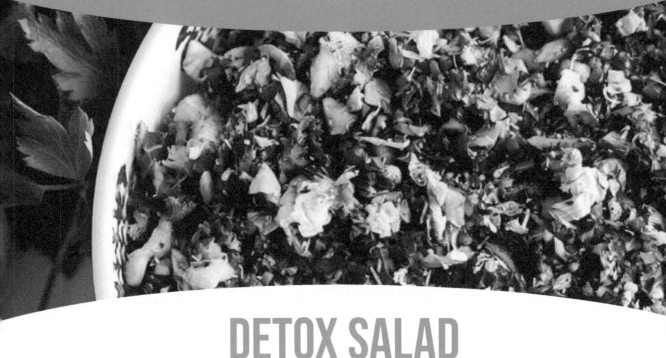

DETOX SALAD

INGREDIENTS

Detox Salad

3 large beets, peeled and shredded

½ head green cabbage, finely chopped

1 bunch dinosaur kale, de-stemmed and shredded

½ C fresh cilantro, finely chopped

Zest of 1 lemon

Detox Salad Dressing

2 lemons, juiced

⅓ C sun butter

1 Tbsp fresh ginger, grated

4 Tbsp raw unfiltered apple cider vinegar

DIRECTIONS

Detox Salad

Combine all the ingredients in a large mixing bowl.

Detox Salad Dressing

Combine all ingredients in a food processor or blender and blend for 1-2 minutes, or until smooth and creamy.

Toss the salad ingredients with the dressing. Plate and top off with a generous sprinkling of the fresh lemon zest.

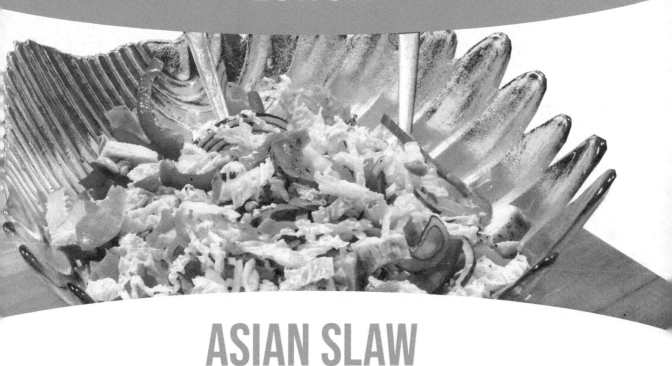

ASIAN SLAW

INGREDIENTS

1 small head shredded green or white cabbage

2 large carrots, peeled and grated

1 red bell pepper, thinly sliced

1 C cooked and shelled edamame

2 medium scallions, finely sliced

½ C chopped or whole salted peanuts

½ C loosely packed fresh cilantro, chopped

DIRECTIONS

In a large bowl, combine all ingredients and mix.

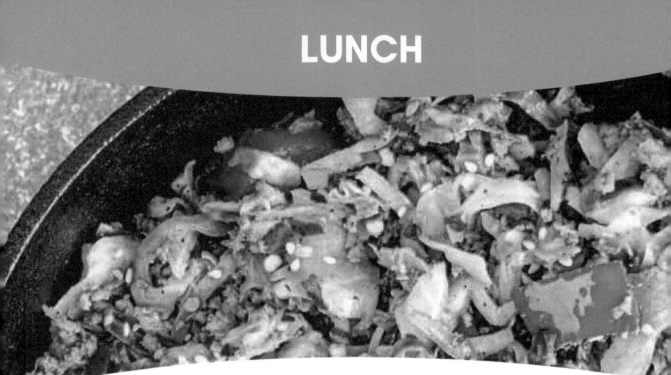

CRACK SLAW

INGREDIENTS

1 lb ground beef
2 Tbsp toasted sesame oil
2 minced garlic cloves
3 sliced green onions
14 oz coleslaw mix
Sea salt/ground black pepper to taste

DIRECTIONS

Brown the ground beef in a skillet and season it with salt and pepper to taste. While the meat is browning combine hot sauce, soy sauce, sweetener, vinegar and ginger. Remove the beef from the pan and set aside. Drain off the fat. Heat up the sesame oil and sauté the garlic, onions and coleslaw mix, until the cabbage is cooked to the desired tenderness. Stir in the sauce. Add the ground beef in and mix well to combine. For the sauce, stir in ¼ tsp white sugar or sweetener, ½ tsp ginger paste, 1 tsp white vinegar, 2 Tbsp soy sauce and chili paste.

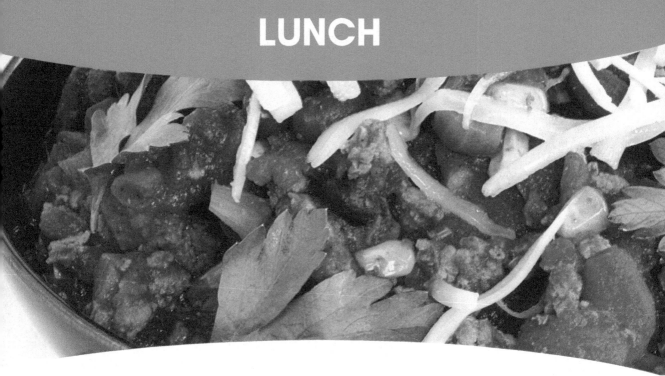

SLOW COOKER TURKEY CHILI

INGREDIENTS

24 oz ground turkey

1 C chopped peppers (I used 1 red, 1 orange, 1 yellow)

1½ C chopped carrots

1 C chopped zucchini (**keep off to the side and add in once the chili is cooked otherwise it will cook too quickly)

28 oz can of chopped tomatoes or tomato sauce

2 Tbsp paprika

1 tsp hot pepper flakes

1 tsp pepper

2 tsp chili powder

1 tsp cumin

1 tsp salt

DIRECTIONS

In a sauce pan brown all of the turkey. Add browned turkey to crock pot. Add in all of the remaining ingredients except for the zucchini. Stir all of the ingredients together until thoroughly mixed.

Cook in the crock pot on high for 3-4 hours. Stirring occasionally. Add in zucchini 5 minutes before serving.

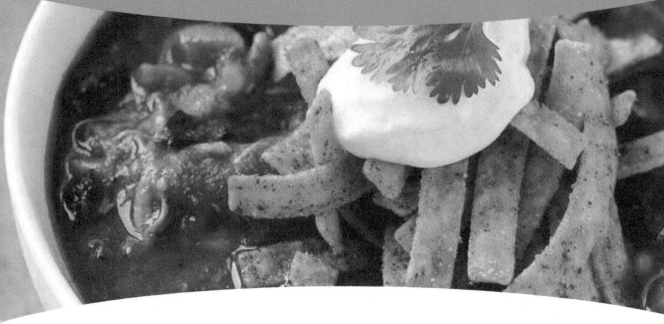

CHICKEN ENCHILADA SOUP

INGREDIENTS

½ C vegetable oil
¼ C chicken stock
3 C diced yellow onions
2 tsp ground cumin
2 tsp chili powder
2 tsp granulated garlic
½ tsp cayenne pepper
2 C masa harina
4 quarts of water
2 C crushed tomatoes
½ lb processed American cheese, small cubes
3 lb cooked, cubed chicken

DIRECTIONS

In a large pot, place oil, chicken base, onion and spices (cumin to cayenne pepper). Saute until onions are soft and clear, about 5 minutes. In another container, combine masa harina with 1 quart of water. Stir until all lumps dissolve. Add to sautéed onions and bring to boil. Once mixture starts to bubble, continue cooking 2-3 minutes, stirring constantly. This will eliminate any raw taste from masa harina. Add remaining 3 quarts water to pot. Add tomatoes; let mixture return to boil sirring occasionally. Add cheese to soup. Cook stirring occasionally, until cheese melts. Add chicken; heat through.

GRILLED CHEESE CAULIFLOWER SANDWICHES

INGREDIENTS

1 head riced cauliflower

1 egg beaten

1½ C cheddar or edam cheese, grated

12 slices mozzarella cheese

1½ C queso de bola

⅛ tsp dried sage

⅛ tsp dried oregano

Dash tsp ground mustard seed

Dash tsp dried thyme

Ground black pepper

Butter for greasing

Fresh parsley for garnishing

DIRECTIONS

Strain excess liquid of riced cauliflower. Combine riced cauliflower, beaten egg and ½ C of the grated cheese in a bowl then sprinkle some pepper, mustard seed, sage, oregano and thyme. Mix well. In a slightly greased baking sheet, form cauliflower mixture to resemble a slice of bread. This recipe made 4 slices, about 1 inch thick for each slice. More slices for thinner pieces. Bake cauliflower slices for about 10 to 12 minutes. In a skillet, melt butter at low heat and lay one slice of cauliflower "bread," cover with slices of mozzarella cheese, sprinkle with the grated queso de bola, then top with slices of mozzarella cheese and cover with another slice of cauliflower "bread." Cover skillet and watch closely as mozzarella cheese melts over low heat. Occasionally check the bottom side to avoid burning. If the heat may seem too low, turn to medium heat but move the queso de bola cauliflower "bread" at the sides then cover the skillet again. Flip to the other side and continue to melt mozzarella cheese. Edam cheese doesn't melt quickly so it will just blend with the melted mozzarella cheese. Use a multi-serving wide flat/wide-slotted tongs to safely flip the cauliflower sandwich. Once mozzarella has melted to your desired consistency, place on a plate, garnish with parsley and enjoy!

TURKEY CUCUMBER ROLL

INGREDIENTS

1 cucumber

½ C veggie dip

2 slices turkey deli meat

DIRECTIONS

Use your veggie peeler to create long "Noodles" with the cucumber. Take two noodles and overlap them to form one large noodle. Spread about 1 Tbsp of veggie dip on the cucumber slices then add ¼ slice of turkey meat. Cut cucumber noodles in half then roll each half up.

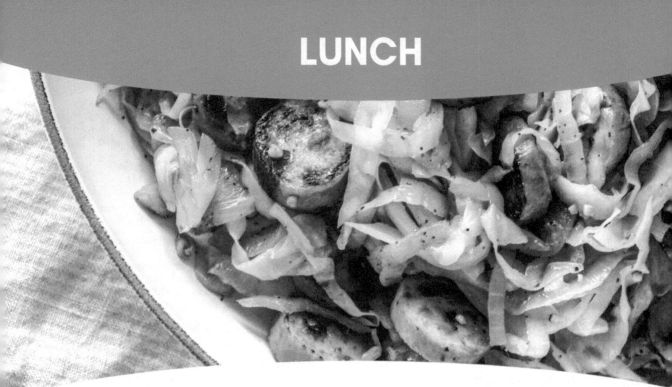

SAUSAGE AND CABBAGE

INGREDIENTS

6 chicken sausage, 1 pound
2 lbs cabbage
4 strips raw bacon
4 oz onion, sliced thinly
1 clove garlic, chopped
Sea salt/ground black pepper to taste

DIRECTIONS

Grill the sausage. Cut the cabbage in half (from top to bottom) and then into quarters. Cut out the core of the cabbage on each quarter. Cut the cabbage quarters into thin strips as if you were making coleslaw. Chop the bacon into small pieces. Cook the bacon in a frying pan until crispy. Add the onion and garlic to the bacon and sauté until softened. Add the sliced cabbage and sauté until it is wilted and cooked down. It will take a while and you may have to add the cabbage in batches. While the cabbage is cooking, slice the sausage into bite-sized pieces. When the cabbage is just about cooked through, add the sausage to warm it through. Add salt and pepper to taste.

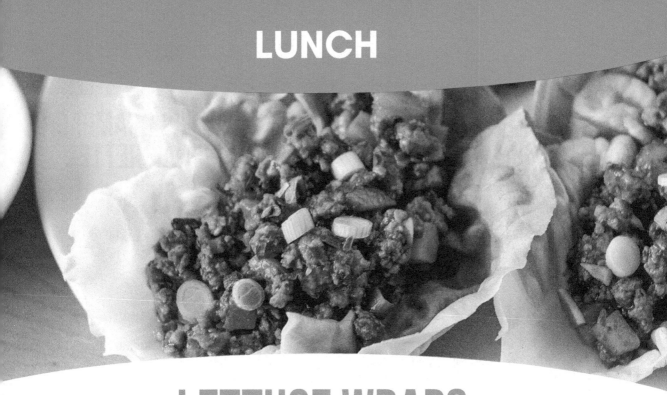

LETTUCE WRAPS

INGREDIENTS

1 tsp sesame oil
2 tsp peanut oil
1 tsp garlic chopped
1 tsp ginger chopped
1 lb ground chicken
1 can chopped water chestnuts
¼ C gluten-free soy sauce (tamari)
1 tsp corn starch
3 tsp honey
2 tsp rice vinegar
3 tsp mirin

DIRECTIONS

Heat oils and sauté garlic and ginger. Add ground chicken to pan and cook till no longer pink. Drain off grease and add water chestnuts to the pan. Into separate bowl mix together ¼ C gluten-free soy sauce. Pour over the chicken mixture, reserve 1 Tbsp of the grease with a tsp of corn starch and add it back to thicken.

Serve with bibb or hydroponic lettuce, shredded carrots, Sriracha, and jasmine rice. For extra crunch, I will sometimes fry white rice noodles in vegetable oil and sprinkle for on top.

DRESSINGS

KALE PESTO DRESSING

INGREDIENTS

2 to 3 cloves garlic
3 C packed kale (about 1 small bunch)
¾ C hemp seeds or toasted walnuts or pecans
2 Tbsp lemon juice (about 1 lemon)
¾ tsp fine-grain sea salt
¼ tsp ground pepper
Red pepper flakes, optional (if you want to add some kick)
¼ C flaxseed oil or extra-virgin olive oil (more if desired)

CILANTRO CHAMPAGNE VINAIGRETTE

INGREDIENTS

1 garlic clove, finely chopped
½ Tbsp Dijon mustard
¼ C champagne vinegar
2 Tbsp fresh lemon juice
2 Tbsp honey
½ tsp salt
½ tsp freshly ground black pepper
½ C extra virgin olive oil
1 C cilantro

CREAMY VEGAN CAESAR DRESSING

INGREDIENTS

1 Tbsp Dijon mustard
2 Tbsp nutritional yeast
½ C vegan mayonnaise
1 tsp crushed garlic
2 tsp capers
2 Tbsp lemon juice
1 Tbsp gluten free soy sauce*
1 Tbsp maple syrup
1 Tbsp extra virgin olive oil
¼ tsp white vinegar

CREAMY AVOCADO ARTICHOKE PESTO DRESSING

INGREDIENTS

2 avocados
2 C basil
¼ C cashews
½ lemon, juiced
2 garlic cloves
⅛ tsp salt and pepper
2 C water

DIRECTIONS:
For all dressings

Add all ingredients into a high speed blender or food processor. Scrape down sides to make sure all the ingredients are mixed until smooth. Add a Tbsp of water a time if needed until you've reached your desired consistency.

DINNER RECIPES

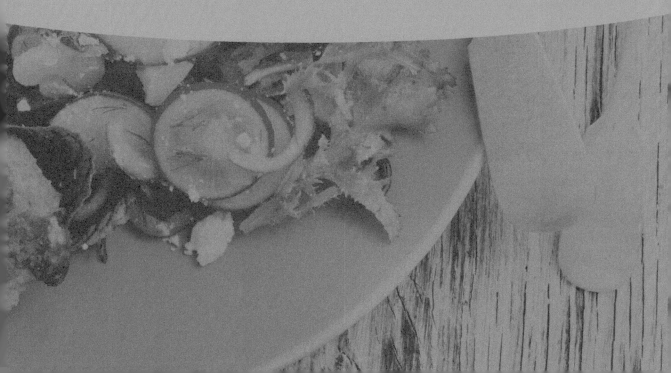

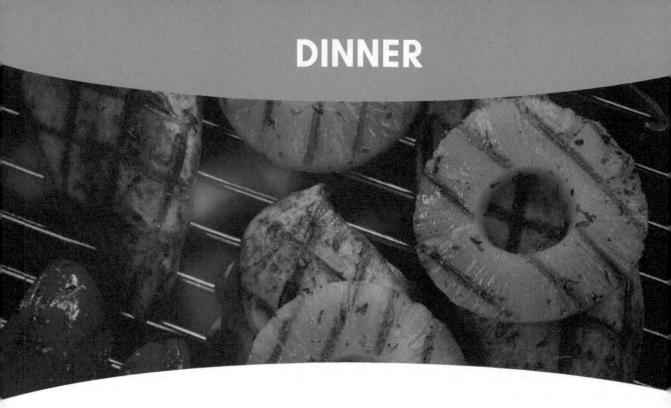

GRILLED PINEAPPLE CHICKEN

INGREDIENTS

4 chicken breasts, skinless, boneless
1 zucchini, sliced
1 bell pepper, chopped
1 pineapple, peeled and sliced
1 red onion, sliced

Teriyaki-style sauce
½ C coconut aminos
2 Tbsp white wine vinegar
Juice of 1 lemon
¼ C fresh pineapple juice
¾ tsp. Ground ginger

DIRECTIONS

In a saucepan, combine all the ingredients for the teriyaki sauce and season to taste. Bring to a boil over medium-high heat, lower the heat and let simmer for 5 to 6 minutes. Rub the chicken with ¼ of the teriyaki sauce, and let marinate 30 minutes. Preheat a grill to medium-high. Grill the chicken breasts for 5 to 8 minutes per side. Place the vegetables in a grill basket and grill until soft, 4 to 5 minutes. Grill the pineapple for 3 minutes per side. Slice the chicken breasts and pineapple, and serve on top of a bed of vegetables, with the remaining teriyaki sauce.

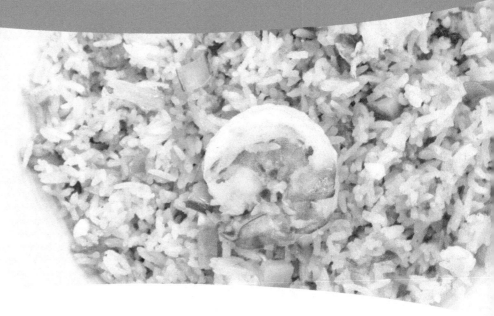

CAULIFLOWER SHRIMP FRIED RICE

INGREDIENTS

2 Tbsp coconut oil

8 oz raw peeled shrimp

Pinch of sea salt

1 stem lemongrass, finely chopped

½ long red chili, finely chopped

½ red or white onion, finely diced

1 large carrot, diced into small cubes

1 celery stick, diced into small cubes

1 medium head of cauliflower, finely diced

2 large cloves of garlic, finely diced

1 Tbsp fish sauce

2 Tbsp coconut aminos

Generous pinch of sea salt

1 tsp sesame oil

1 Tbsp lime juice

Handful of cilantro leaves, chopped

DIRECTIONS

Heat 1 Tbsp of coconut oil in a large frying pan over high heat and add the shrimp. Sprinkle with a little sea salt and stir-fry for 2-3 minutes, until the shrimp curl and change color. Transfer to a bowl. Reduce the heat to medium-high and add 1 Tbsp of coconut oil. Add the lemon grass, chili, onions, carrots and celery and stir-fry for 3 minutes, until softened and fragrant. Now add the finely diced cauliflower and the rest of the ingredients and stir-fry for 2-3 minutes. Add a few Tbsp of water if the frying pan gets dry. Stir in the shrimp right at the end to reheat and top with fresh cilantro.

ONE MEAL AND A TASTING

137

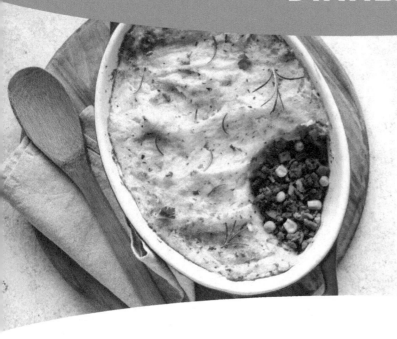

SHEPHERD'S PIE

INGREDIENTS

1¼ lbs ground beef
½ medium onion, chopped
5 large garlic cloves, minced
1 medium carrot, shredded
1 medium zucchini, shredded
1 Tbsp olive oil
1½ tsp salt
1 tsp chili powder

Mashed Cauliflower Recipe
2 small cauliflower heads
7 large roasted garlic cloves
1 tsp salt

DIRECTIONS

Heat the olive oil in a large skillet over medium heat, and sauté the onion and garlic until tender. Add the carrot and zucchini, and cook until they start to soften. Add the ground beef, salt, and chili powder, and cook until the beef browns and all of the moisture begins to dry out. Meanwhile prepare the mashed cauliflower. Chop the cauliflower heads into small chunks, and steam until they soften (a fork can easily pierce). Add the steamed cauliflower, roasted garlic and salt to a blender and blend until you have a smooth pureé. Use the tamper to help blend the cauliflower if you have one. To assemble the pie, distribute the ground beef evenly in the bottom of an 8-inch baking dish. Spread the mashed cauliflower over the top of the ground beef, and bake in a preheated oven to 350° for 25 minutes. If you're adding cheese (I use mozzarella) to the top of your shepherd's pie, sprinkle the cheese on top after you bake it, and then broil it until the cheese browns.

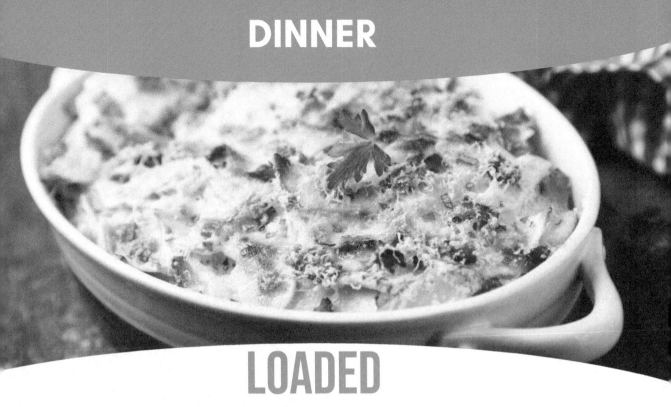

LOADED CAULIFLOWER CHICKEN CASSEROLE

INGREDIENTS

1 lbs chicken breasts
4 C of cauliflower, cubed
¼ C olive oil
1 tsp pepper
1 Tbsp garlic powder
3 Tbsp hot sauce

Toppings:
1 C fiesta Mexican blend cheese
½ C crumbled cooked bacon
½ C diced green onion

DIRECTIONS

Preheat oven to 500°. In a large bowl mix together the olive oil, hot sauce, salt, pepper, garlic powder and paprika. Add the cubed cauliflower and stir to coat. Add the cauliflower to a greased baking dish. When scooping the cauliflower into the baking dish, leave behind any extra olive oil/hot sauce mix. Add the diced chicken to the "left behind" olive oil/hot sauce mix and stir to coat all the chicken. Allow to marinate as the cauliflower bakes. Roast the cauliflower for 40-50 minutes, stirring every 10-15 minutes, until cooked through and nice and crispy on the outside. Once the cauliflower is fully cooked, remove from the oven, add the marinated chicken, and lower the oven temperature to 400°. In a large bowl mix all the topping ingredients together. Top the chicken with the topping. Bake 15 minutes or until the chicken is cooked through and the topping is melted and bubbly delicious.

TOM JONES SHRIMP

INGREDIENTS

1 lb. Shrimp
1 Tbsp pepper
1½ tsp salt
Juice of 1 lemon
1 Tbsp Worcestershire sauce
Hot sauce
1 clove of garlic crushed
3 Tbsp olive oil
3 Tbsp butter, melted

DIRECTIONS

Mix together all ingredients, spread on baking sheet and bake at 350° for 20 min. or until shrimp is cooked.

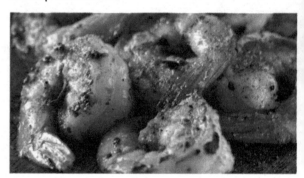

MEATBALLS

INGREDIENTS

1 lb grass-fed ground beef
1 lb ground turkey (check for no added ingredients)
1 large egg, room temperature
2 Tbsp Italian seasoning
½ tsp salt
½ C almond flour
2 Tbsp coconut amino

DIRECTIONS

Preheat the oven to 400° and line a sheet tray with parchment paper.

In a large bowl, combine beef, turkey, egg, Italian seasoning, salt, almond flour, and coconut aminos. Mix until everything is completely combined. The best way to do that is with clean hands. Wash your hands, then use a cookie scoop to make balls. Roll between palms to make smooth. Place on prepared sheet tray and bake for 20 minutes.

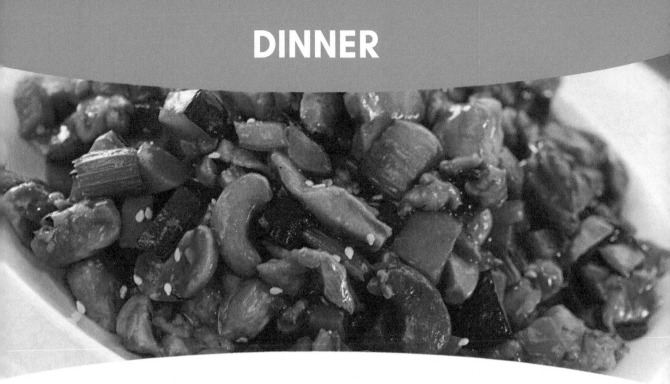

CASHEW CHICKEN

INGREDIENTS

3 raw chicken thighs boneless, skinless
2 Tbsp canola oil (for cooking)
¼ C cashews
½ medium green bell pepper
½ tsp ground ginger
1 Tbsp rice wine vinegar
1½ Tbsp soy sauce
½ Tbsp chili garlic sauce
1 Tbsp minced garlic
1 Tbsp sesame oil
1 Tbsp sesame seeds
1 Tbsp green onions
¼ medium white onion
Sea salt/ground black pepper to taste

DIRECTIONS

Heat a pan over low heat and toast the cashews for 8 minutes or until they start to lightly brown and become fragrant. Remove and set aside. Dice chicken thighs into 1 inch chunks. Cut onion and pepper into equally large chunks. Increase heat to high and add canola oil to pan. Once oil is up to temperature, add in the chicken thighs and allow them to cook through (about 5 minutes). Once the chicken is fully cooked. Add in the pepper, onions, garlic, chili garlic sauce and seasonings (ginger, salt, pepper). Allow to cook on high for 2-3 minutes. Add soy sauce, rice wine vinegar, and cashews. Cook on high and allow the liquid to reduce down until it is a sticky consistency, there should not be excess liquid in the pan upon completing cooking. Serve in a bowl, top with sesame seeds and green onions and drizzle with sesame oil.

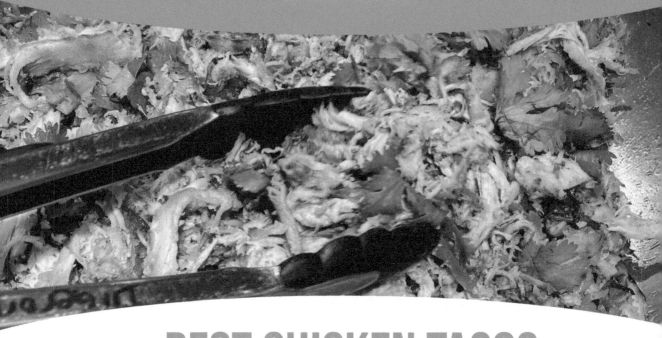

BEST CHICKEN TACOS

INGREDIENTS

2 Tbsp Avocado oil
2 onions, sliced super skinny
1 roasted chicken
4 cloves of garlic
1 tsp cumin
4 Tbsp fresh cilantro
3 tsp honey
2 Tbsp organic butter

DIRECTIONS

Buy a roasted chicken. Shred all chicken off the roasted chicken. Separate dark meat and white in a separate containers.

Lightly brown avocado oil and sliced onions in a pan. Add some more avocado oil and garlic. Add pulled chicken off rotisserie. Then, sear the chicken and add 4 cloves of garlic and 1 tsp cumin.

At the end add 4 Tbsp fresh cilantro, 3 tsp honey, 2 Tbsp organic butter and garnish at the end with ½ C of cilantro and 2 limes.

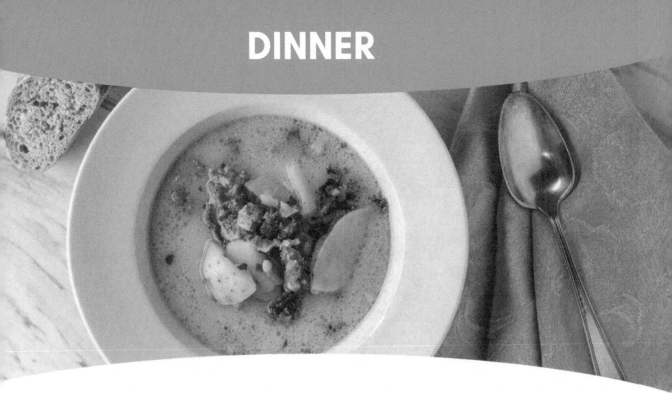

SLOW COOKER ZUPPA TOSCANA

INGREDIENTS

1 lb. organic spicy chicken sausage
1 head cauliflower, cut into small florets
1 onion, chopped
¼ C real bacon pieces
2 Tbsp minced garlic (about 3 or 4 cloves)
32 oz. Chicken broth
1 C kale chopped

DIRECTIONS

Brown sausage links in sauté pan. Cut links in half lengthwise, then cut slices. Place sausage, chicken broth, garlic, cauliflower and onion in slow cooker. Add just enough water to cover the vegetables and meat.

Cook on high 3-4 hours (low 5-6 hours). 30 minutes before serving mix flour into cream removing lumps. Add cream, kale and bacon to the crock pot, stir. Cook on high 30 minutes or until broth thickens slightly. Add salt, pepper and cayenne to taste.

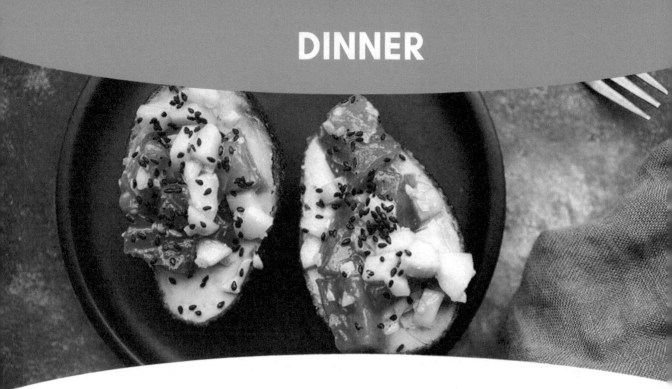

TUNA POKE AVOCADO BOATS

INGREDIENTS

1 lb sushi-grade tuna, diced

¼ C coconut aminos (plus more for serving)

1 Tbsp toasted sesame oil

1 cucumber, seeds removed and diced

3 Tbsp macadamia nuts, chopped

8 avocados, halved

1 Tbsp black sesame seeds, for garnish (optional)

DIRECTIONS

In a large bowl, combine diced tuna, coconut aminos and toasted sesame oil and combine well. Place in the fridge while you chop the cucumber and macadamias to allow the fish to marinate a bit. Once the cucumber and nuts are chopped, add to the bowl with the tuna. If you don't plan on serving this right away, cover and keep fish in the fridge. When you are ready to eat, halve two avocados and place a bit of the fish into the hole of each. Top with a sprinkling of black sesame seeds.

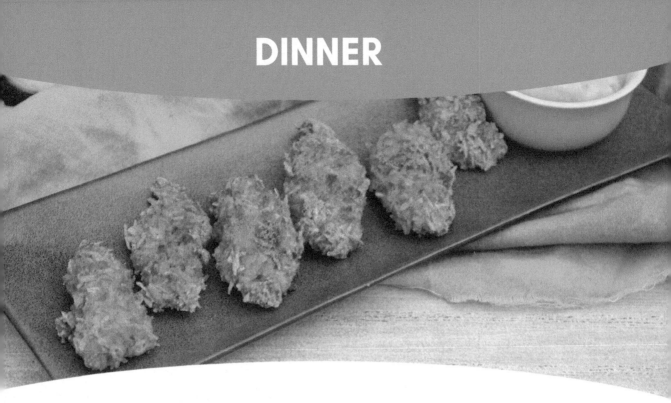

CHICKEN TENDERS

INGREDIENTS

1 egg

½ C almond meal

¼ C unsweetened shredded coconut

1 tsp paprika

½ tsp cayenne pepper

½ tsp garlic powder

½ tsp sea salt

¼ tsp black pepper

1 egg

1 lb organic boneless skinless chicken breast, cut into strips

DIRECTIONS

Preheat oven to 400°. Place almond meal, coconut, paprika, cayenne, garlic, sea salt and black pepper in a small bowl. Stir to combine. Crack egg into another shallow bowl and whisk. One by one, dredge each chicken tender in the egg bowl, wiping off any access and then dip each into the almond meal mixture. Roll until each tender is covered completely. Place the coated tenders on a baking pan lined with parchment paper or a wire rack that fits on a baking sheet. The wire rack will make for a crispier texture. Bake for 20 minutes, flipping the tenders once at the 10-minute mark. When done, the chicken tenders will be golden brown and completely cooked through. Remove tenders from the oven and allow to cool slightly before serving.

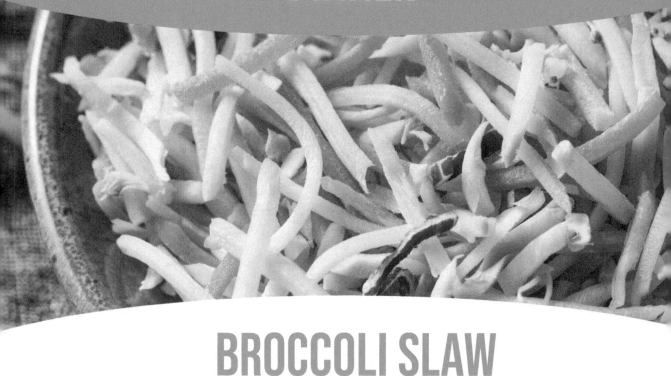

BROCCOLI SLAW

INGREDIENTS

2 packages broccoli cole slaw (12 oz each)
½ C diced sweet vidalia onions
½ C olive oil
½ C cider vinegar
½ tsp black pepper
1 tsp dill weed
½ tsp celery seed
½ tsp salt
¼ tsp turmeric
¼ tsp onion powder
¼ tsp garlic powder
¼ tsp paprika
1 C sliced almonds

DIRECTIONS

Place the broccoli cole slaw in a large bowl. Add the onions and mix. Set aside. In a small bowl or shaker C, combine the olive oil, vinegar and spices. Stir or shake well. Pour the dressing over the cole slaw and stir to coat. Just before serving, mix in the sliced almonds.

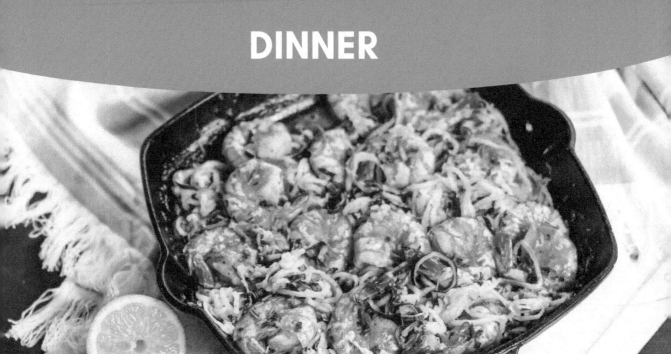

LEMON GARLIC SHRIMP

INGREDIENTS

8 oz raw shrimp, peeled and de-veined, tail left on
1 tsp seafood seasoning
2 Tbsp avocado oil
2 garlic cloves, finely chopped
1 Tbsp lemon juice
1 Tbsp chopped fresh parsley

DIRECTIONS

In a small bowl, toss shrimp with seafood seasoning and set aside. Heat avocado oil in a large skillet over medium high heat. Add garlic and sauté until fragrant. Add the shrimp and cook until pink, stirring frequently, about 5 minutes. Add lemon juice and fresh parsley and toss to combine.

Remove shrimp from pan and set aside. Add cauliflower rice (page 61) for a delicious dinner.

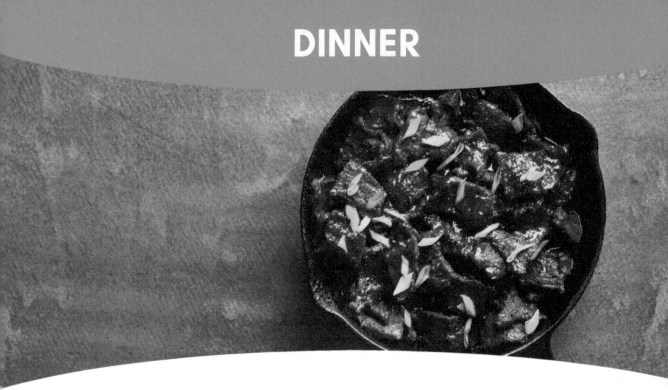

MONGOLIAN BEEF

INGREDIENTS

1 lb. flank steak

3 Tbsp arrowroot flour

½ tsp sea salt

½ tsp ground pepper

1 Tbsp + ½ C lard/bacon fat or tallow

2 cloves garlic, minced

1 tsp dried ginger

Dash red pepper flakes (optional)

1 Tbsp toasted sesame oil

½ C coconut amino's

½ C chicken or beef broth

⅓ C raw honey

3 green onions, chopped

DIRECTIONS

Cut the flank steak against the grain into ⅓ inch slices. In a medium-sized bowl mix together the arrowroot flour, pepper, and salt. Dip each piece of steak into the arrowroot flour and shake off any excess coating. Lay coated steak on a drying rack and allow to sit for 10-15 minutes. This allows the powder to adhere to the steak better. While your steak is hanging out, you can make the sauce. Heat the 1 Tbsp of lard/ bacon fat or tallow in a medium-sized saucepan over medium heat. Add the garlic, ginger and dash of red pepper flakes (optional) and cook for about 1 minute. Add the sesame oil, coconut aminos and broth to the pan and stir ingredients together. Add the raw honey and allow it to melt into the sauce, stirring frequently. Turn the heat up to high and continue to stir until the sauce thickens slightly, about 3 minutes. Turn off the sauce and allow it to sit in the pan while you cook the steak. Add your ½ C of your favorite fat to a large skillet. Cook over medium heat until hot. Gently drop the beef into the oil using your tongs. Cook for 2-3 minutes until lightly browned around the edges. Remove the beef with tongs and place on a paper towel-lined plate. Pour out the oil from the pan and add the beef back in. Cook for about 1 minute and then add the sauce. Cook together for about 3 minutes, then add the green onions and cook for 1 additional minute. Remove the beef from the pan and pour any excess sauce into a bowl.

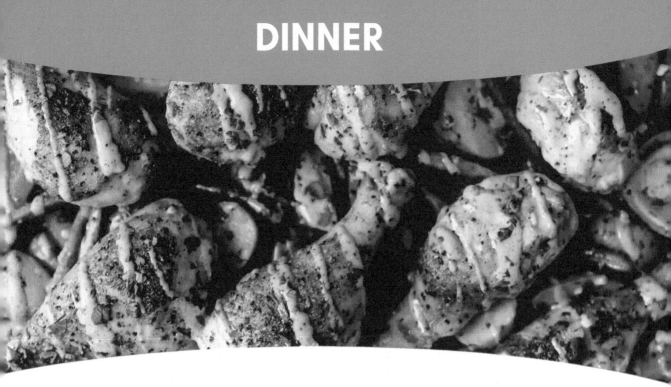

ONE-PAN CHICKEN CAESAR VEGGIE BAKE

INGREDIENTS

2 lbs of chicken legs, skin on
(Can sub for thighs or breasts)
¾ C Caesar dressing
16 oz cauliflower, chopped
12 oz carrots, cut into 2-3 inch sticks
12 oz green beans, trimmed
3-4 cloves garlic, minced (2 Tbsp.)
½ Tbsp Avocado or olive oil
Sea salt/ground black pepper to taste

DIRECTIONS

Place the Caesar dressing and chicken legs in a glass container. Toss to coat. Cover and refrigerate. Marinate for at least 4 hours or overnight.

Preheat oven to 425°. Line a large baking sheet with parchment (optional). Add veggies to the pan, drizzle lightly with oil, toss to coat veggies. Make spaces for chicken legs. Remove chicken legs from marinade and add to pan. Discard excess marinade. Dash all with salt and pepper.

Bake in the oven for 20 minutes. Remove from oven and toss veggies and flip chicken legs. Place pan back in oven and bake for an additional 8-10 minutes. Remove from oven and serve. Drizzle chicken and veggies with a little Caesar dressing if you wish. Garnish with chopped parsley and cracked black pepper.

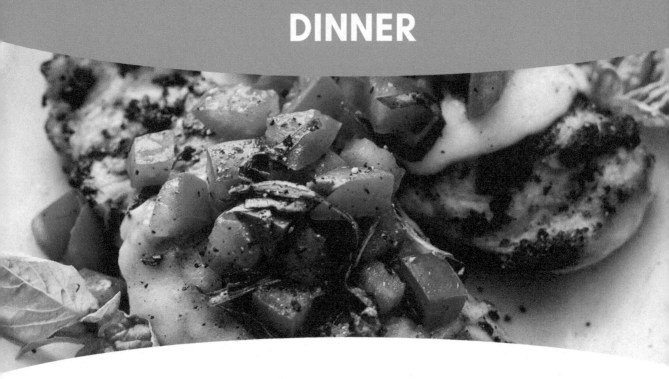

HEALTHY BRUSCHETTA CHICKEN

INGREDIENTS

Chicken:
2 Tbsp. Olive oil, extra virgin
4 chicken breasts
Salt & Pepper to taste
1 Tbsp. dried basil
1 Tbsp. Minced Garlic

Bruschetta:
3 ripe Roma tomatoes, diced
7 basil leaves, chopped
1 sprig oregano, chopped
2 tsp minced garlic
1 Tbsp. olive oil, extra virgin
1 tsp balsamic vinegar
¼ tsp Salt
¼ tsp Pepper

Balsamic Glaze:
1 C Balsamic Vinegar

DIRECTIONS

Chicken:
Add olive oil to sauté pan or cast-iron skillet. Heat pan to medium high heat. Add chicken to hot pan. Sprinkle salt, pepper, and dried basil on top of each cutlet. Cook until browned, about 5 minutes. Flip chicken. Add garlic to the pan. Cook until remaining side of chicken is browned, about 5 minutes

Bruschetta:
Add all ingredients to a bowl and stir together until combined. Pour over your cooked chicken breasts

Balsamic Glaze:
Add 1 C of balsamic vinegar to a small saucepan. Bring to a boil over medium high heat. Reduce heat to medium. You will see bubbling along the outside of your pan. Let simmer for 10 minutes. Stir occasionally as vinegar begins to thicken and coat the spoon. Remove from heat and allow to cook for a few minutes. Sauce will thicken more as it sits, you will end up with ¼ C of balsamic glaze. Drizzle over bruschetta-topped chicken.

SIZZLIN' BEEF ROAST

INGREDIENTS

1 beef shoulder
2 C of baby carrots
4-5 stalks of celery
1 white onion
1 tsp garlic
2 tsps salt
1 tsp pepper

For Sauce
¼ C butter
2 Tbsp gluten-free flour

DIRECTIONS

Add all ingredients into a pan and fill it ¾ of the way up. Oven set at 300° for 7 hours.
To make sauce, take butter, gluten-free flour and beef broth to put on top of beef.

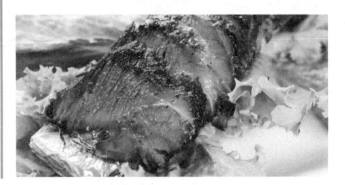

CAULIFLOWER RICE

INGREDIENTS

2 tsp avocado oil
2 garlic cloves, finely chopped
1 tsp fresh grated ginger
3 green onions, chopped
1 large bell pepper, seeded and diced
1 lb riced cauliflower (frozen is okay)
2 C finely chopped kale
3 Tbsp coconut aminos
1 tsp sea salt
¼ tsp crushed red pepper flakes
1 C heavy whipping cream
2 tsp corn starch

DIRECTIONS

Add avocado oil to the same skillet you used for the shrimp (page 57), and turn the heat up a bit. Add the garlic, ginger and green Onions to oil. Sauté, stirring Frequently, for 1 minute.

Add bell pepper, cauliflower, kale, Coconut aminos, salt and pepper flakes. Stir-fry until veggies are Tender, about 5 to 7 minutes. Serve with shrimp, hot sauce and extra Coconut aminos if desired.

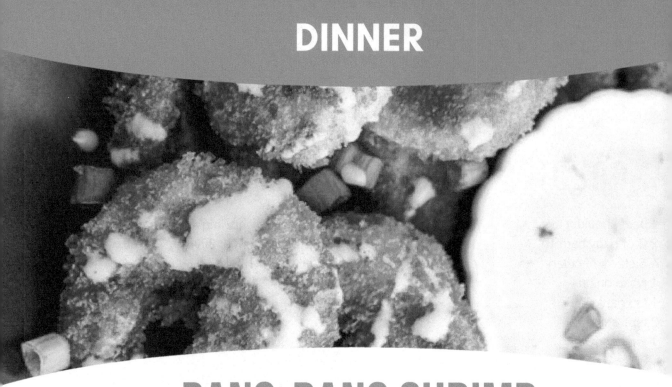

BANG-BANG SHRIMP

INGREDIENTS

1 head iceberg lettuce
3 Tbsp Thai sweet chili sauce
⅓ C mayonnaise
1 Tbsp Sriracha hot sauce
1 lb raw wild caught shrimp
¾ C arrowroot starch
1 tsp seasoned salt
4 C lard
Onion powder
Garlic powder

DIRECTIONS

Thaw frozen shrimp in a bowl of cool water. Combine mayo, chili sauce and Sriracha hot sauce in a small bowl. Put in the fridge to chill while you're preparing everything else. Prepare your oil for frying either in a pot on the stove or in a separate deep fryer. Heat oil to 350°. Line a plate with paper towel, to drain fried shrimp. Peel off the shells and remove tail. Butterfly your shrimp by cutting down the back but not all the way through. Allow them to drain in a colander. Put the arrowroot starch in a bag or bowl, season lightly with sea salt, pepper, onion and garlic powder. Toss shrimp in the seasoned arrowroot powder, until lightly coated. Using your hands to scoop out the cornstarch-dusted shrimp, gently shake off excess. Carefully drop shrimp into the 350° oil, fry for 1-2 minutes and drain on paper towel. Pile up some lettuce on your dinner plate, add shrimp and drizzle with sauce.

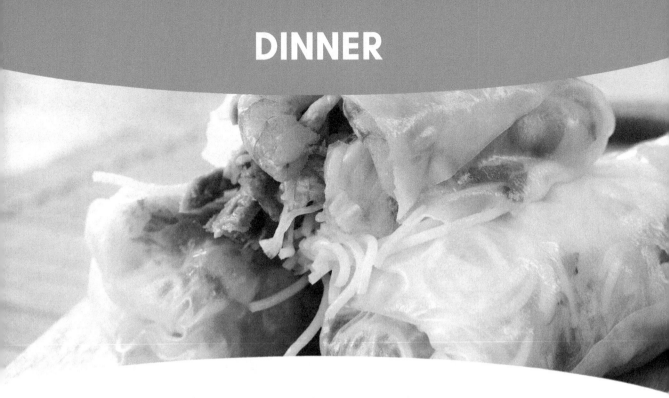

SPRING ROLLS

INGREDIENTS

1 package of rice paper

6-7 medium-sized raw shrimp (about ¼ lb)

1 carrot, thinly sliced

½ cucumber, seeds removed and thinly sliced

2 green onions, dark green tops removed and thinly sliced

1 bunch of fresh mint, basil or cilantro leaves

6 oz kelp noodles, optional

¼ C of umami mayo for dipping, optional

DIRECTIONS

Set up a large bowl with ice water. Bring a very large pot of water to boiling. Dip the whole collard leaves in the boiling water for 1 minute. Immediately place them in the ice water to cool and stop the cooking process. Drain and set aside. Peel and de-vein the shrimp, if needed. Into a small skillet over medium heat, place the raw shrimp and 2-3 Tbsp of water. Cover and steam until the shrimp are pink, about 2 Minutes. Set aside to cool. Slice in half from head to tail. Rinse and drain the kelp noodles. Set aside. Prepare the carrot, cucumber and green onion. How thinly you slice them depends on how much chewing you want to be involved. Now assemble a wrap: lay the rice paper on a flat surface. Place two halves of shrimp at the top of the leaf. Next, put a small amount of kelp noodles (a little less than a¼C worked for me) on top of the shrimp. Now you're ready to wrap, burrito-style. Gently but with a bit of pressure, roll from the shrimp-end toward the opposite end. Once you've rolled over once, fold in the sides and then finish rolling all way down. Repeat with the remaining ingredients. Slice each wrap in half and serve cold with your choice of dipping sauces, if desired.

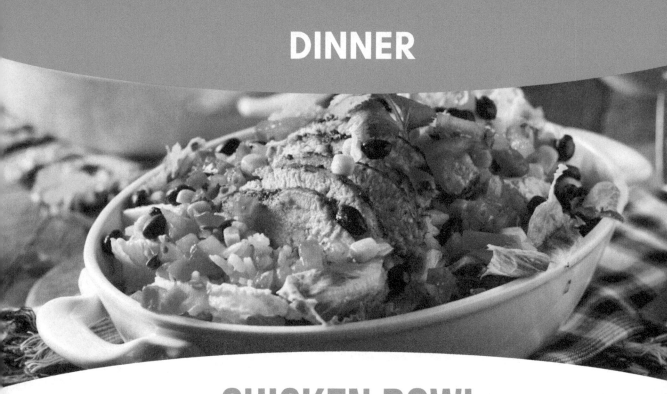

CHICKEN BOWL

INGREDIENTS

2 avocados

12 oz jar of roasted peppers - drained

2 cloves garlic - peeled

1lb boneless skinless chicken thighs

1 Tbsp avocado or olive oil

½ red onion - peeled and diced

2 C mushrooms - sliced

6 C greens (spinach, kale, etc.)

Sea salt/ground black pepper to taste

DIRECTIONS

First make roasted pepper sauce by placing avocado, the peppers, garlic cloves and a pinch of salt and pepper into a food processor. Blend until smooth and place in refrigerator to chill. Season chicken with salt and pepper on both sides. Heat a large skillet over medium heat and add avocado oil. Once hot, add chicken to cook, about 4-5 minutes per side. While the chicken is cooking, cut up onion, mushrooms, and greens. Once the chicken is cooked through, remove from skillet and place on a cooking board to rest. Add onion to skillet and cook for 3-4 minutes, stirring frequently until onions begin to soften. Add mushrooms and cook until they start to soften, another 2-3 minutes. Add greens and cook until they begin to wilt, about 1-2 minutes. Remove from heat. Slice chicken into bite-sized pieces and mix with veggies.

Serve in bowls and top each bowl with ½ avocado and a generous amount of roasted pepper sauce.

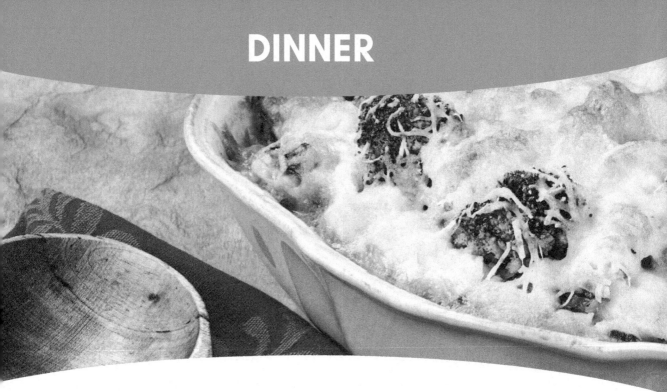

CHEESY BROCCOLI CASSEROLE

INGREDIENTS

30-32 oz (7 C packed) frozen or fresh broccoli florets

1 head cauliflower

1 Tbsp grass-fed butter

1½ C (13.6 oz) full-fat canned coconut milk

2 eggs, lightly beaten

½ C and 2 Tbsp nutritional yeast, divided

1 tsp sea salt

¼ tsp ground black pepper

2 C pork rinds, crushed

DIRECTIONS

Preheat the oven to 350°. Steam the broccoli florets until they're fork-tender. Drain and set aside. Cut the florets from the head of the cauliflower. Either using the grating attachment on your food processor or by simply adding them to the food processor bowl, break them up into rice-sized pieces. Transfer the "rice" to a microwave- safe bowl with a few Tbsp water. Cover and cook for 7 minutes. Drain and set aside. Melt butter in a large frying pan and then add the "rice." Stir well, cover, and let it steam for 5 minutes over medium heat. Remove the lid and continue to stir and cook for an additional 5-10 minutes, or until the rice is cooked. In a large mixing bowl, whisk together the coconut milk, beaten eggs, ½ C nutritional yeast, sea salt, and pepper. Add the cooked broccoli and cauliflower rice. Stir to incorporate. Pour the mixture into a large (9x13") casserole dish. Cover with aluminum foil and bake at 350° for 20 minutes. In a small bowl, mix the 2 C crushed pork rinds with the remaining 2 Tbsp of nutritional yeast. Remove the casserole from the oven and sprinkle the top with the nutritional yeast and pork rind breading. Return to the oven at 350° for an additional 15 minutes. Let cool for 5-10 minutes and then serve warm.

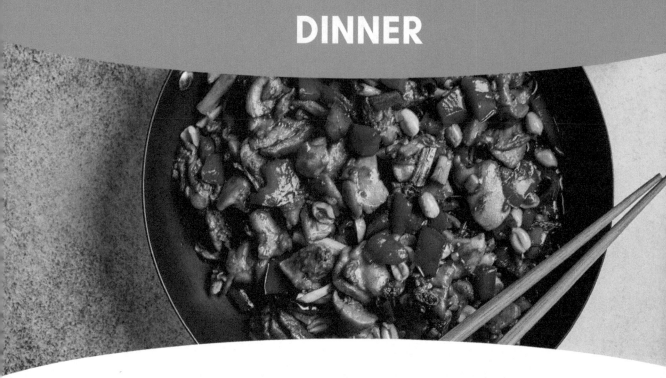

KUNG PAO CHICKEN

INGREDIENTS

1 lb. boneless, skinless chicken thighs
Sea salt
Ground black pepper
2 tsp arrowroot flour
2 tsp sesame oil
3 Tbsp coconut aminos
2 tsp raw honey
½ tsp dried ginger
1 Tbsp lard/bacon fat or tallow
6 small dried red chili peppers, cut in half and
    removed seeds crushed red pepper flakes
    (optional)
2 cloves of garlic, minced
¼ C chopped green onion
⅓ C chopped raw cashews

DIRECTIONS

Cut the chicken thighs into 1 inch pieces and season with sea salt and ground black pepper. Set aside. To make the sauce, place the arrowroot flour, sesame oil and coconut aminos in a small saucepan and stir to combine. Add the raw honey and dried ginger, place over medium heat and bring just to a light boil, stirring frequently. Remove from heat and set aside. In a large skillet or wok, melt the fat over medium-high heat. Add the chili peppers, garlic and a few dashes of red pepper flakes or sichuan peppercorns and sauté for about 30 seconds. Add the chicken and cook 3-5 minutes or until browned on all sides. Add the green onion to the pan and toss to combine. Pour in the sauce and cook for another 2-3 minutes until heated through and the chicken is fully cooked. Add the chopped cashews, stir and serve.

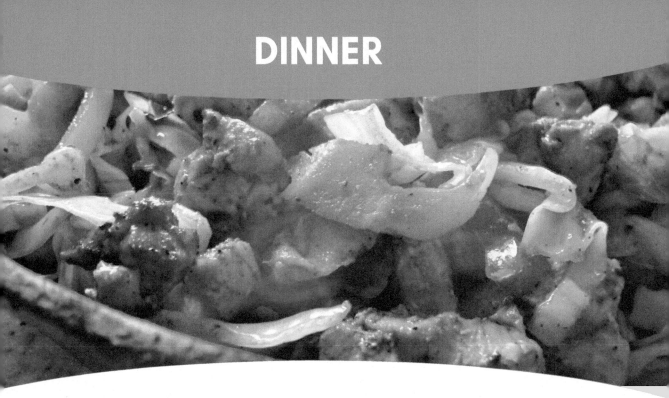

QUICK CHICKEN CABBAGE STIR FRY

INGREDIENTS

1 Tbsp. Coconut Oil

1 lb. chicken breast or thigh meat, sliced into thin strips (bite size)

½ tsp Sea salt

¼ tsp white pepper (can use black pepper, but white is more Asian in flavor)

1 tsp grated ginger

3 C. sliced Napa cabbage (½ medium cabbage)

1 C. broccolini or broccoli florets

1 large carrot, sliced

2 cloves garlic, finely diced

1 tsp fish sauce

3½ Tbsp. coconut aminos
  (can sub 3 Tbsp Tamari sauce)

Juice of ½ a lime (or 2 Tbsp. lemon juice)

1 tsp. Sesame oil

DIRECTIONS

Heat a Tbsp of coconut oil in a large frying pan or a wok over high heat. Once hot, add the chicken and sprinkle with salt and white pepper. Cook for 3 minutes each side and place in a bowl.

Place the pan back over high heat and add another Tbsp coconut oil. Add ginger, cabbage, broccolini and carrots. Cook for 2 minutes, stirring frequently. Add splash of water (about 2 Tbsp.), garlic, fish sauce, coconut aminos, lime juice and return the chicken to the pan. Mix thoroughly and cook for 2 minutes. Drizzle with sesame oil and stir.

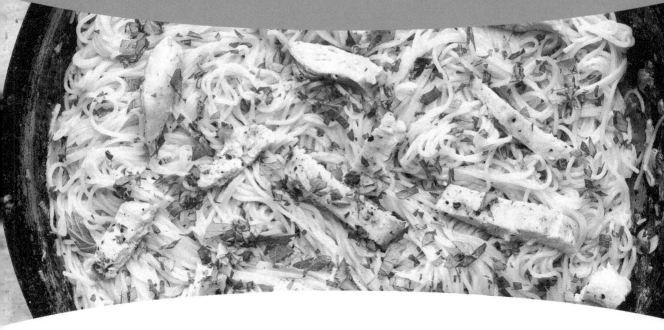

CHICKEN SCAMPI

INGREDIENTS

4 Tbsp unsalted butter divided
½ red bell pepper sliced thinly
½ yellow bell pepper sliced thinly
½ green bell pepper sliced thinly
½ red onion thinly sliced
2 Tbsp garlic minced
4 Tbsp gluten free flour divided
½ tsp red pepper flakes
1 tsp dried oregano
½ tsp dried basil
1 C white wine
1 C chicken broth
1 pound angel hair pasta
1 pound chicken breast tenderloins
1 tsp Kosher salt
½ tsp coarse ground black pepper
2 Tbsp olive oil
½ C heavy cream warm to the touch
½ medium lemon juiced
1 C Parmesan cheese shaved,

DIRECTIONS

Add 2 Tbsp of butter to a cast iron skillet on medium-high heat and cook the bell peppers and onions for 2-3 minutes or until slightly softened. Remove the vegetables and add in remaining 2 Tbsp of butter. Once melted add in 2 Tbsp of flour and garlic. Whisk well until the flour has had a chance to "cook" for about 20 seconds. Add in the red pepper flakes, oregano, basil, wine and chicken broth, then let reduce on medium heat for 18-20 minutes.

While the sauce is reducing cook the pasta one minute shy of the instructions, do not rinse. In a second pan add 2 Tbsp of olive oil on medium high heat. Coat the chicken tenderloins in the salt and pepper before tossing in the remaining flour. Add in the chicken, cooking for 3-4 minutes on each side. Remove the chicken from the heat while the sauce finishes reducing. When the sauce is reduced by half add in the heavy cream and whisk well until you have a nice thick sauce. Add in the lemon juice and half the Parmesan cheese and whisk. Toss with the pasta, bell peppers and onions. Top with the chicken and Parmesan and serve.

DINNER

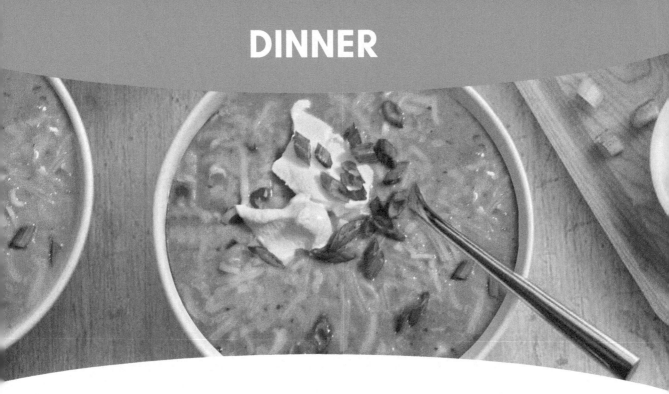

BUFFALO CHICKEN CHILI

INGREDIENTS

Olive oil

Butter

1 lb ground chicken

15 oz canned white navy beans or kidney beans (drained and rinsed)

14½ oz can crushed fire-roasted tomatoes (drained)

2 C chicken broth

¼ - ½ C Buffalo wing sauce (start with ¼ C and add more at end if needed)

1 can of tomato sauce

1 package ranch dressing mix

1 C frozen corn kernels

½ tsp onion powder

½ tsp garlic powder

½ tsp celery salt

½ tsp dried cilantro

½ tsp salt

8 oz cream cheese

DIRECTIONS

Heat olive oil and butter in a large pot over medium-high heat. Place chicken in the pot. Cook and stir 7 to 10 minutes, until chicken is no longer pink. Stir in the carrot, onion, celery, garlic, chili powder, cumin, paprika, and salt and pepper, and cook and stir until the onion is translucent and the vegetables are beginning to soften, 3 to 4 more minutes.

Stir in the buffalo wing sauce, tomato sauce, crushed tomatoes, and white navy beans or red kidney beans. Bring to a boil, and simmer over medium-low heat about 1 hour, until the vegetables are tender and the flavors have blended.

ONE MEAL AND A TASTING

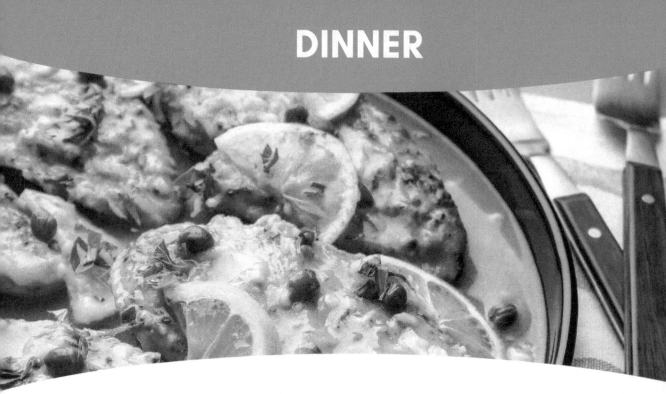

CHICKEN PICCATA

INGREDIENTS

2 large chicken breasts cut in half lengthwise

Sea salt/ground black pepper to taste

1/4 tsp garlic powder

Flour (for dredging)

4 Tbsp butter divided

1 Tbsp olive oil

1/4 C chicken broth or dry white wine

1 Tbsp lemon juice + zest of 1 lemon

1 Tbsp brined capers drained

1/2 C heavy/whipping cream

Garnish (optional) chopped parsley and freshly grated Parmesan cheese

DIRECTIONS

Slice chicken breasts lengthwise (I butterfly then cut in half) to make 4 thinner cutlets. Trim off any fat. Season chicken generously with salt and pepper and sprinkle with garlic powder. Coat the chicken in flour. Add 2 Tbsp of the butter plus the olive oil to a skillet over medium-high heat. Once the pan is hot, cook the chicken pieces for about 4-5 minutes per side until golden. Remove the chicken from skillet and set aside. Take the pan off the heat and add the chicken broth, lemon juice, lemon zest, remaining 2 Tbsp of butter, and capers to the skillet. Scrape up any brown bits. Stir in the cream and return the pan to the heat. Once it's bubbling again, add the chicken back into the pan. If you want to make this recipe without cream, increase the chicken broth to 1/2 C. Cook for another 5 minutes or until the chicken is cooked through and the sauce has reduced to your liking (you may need to turn down the heat a bit if it's bubbling furiously). If the sauce thickens too much, add more broth.

NOTE: After I cooked the chicken, I removed it from the pan and then sautéed the onions and mushrooms in the pan, then followed the recipe from that point. I didn't taste the chicken but I did the cauliflower. I thought is was so good.

Q and A with Chantel Ray

From

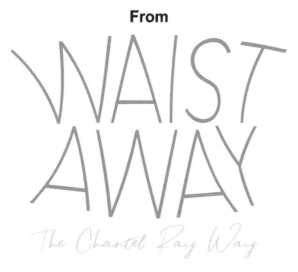

WAIST AWAY

The Chantel Ray Way

Q: **What if I'm plateauing and not losing weight?**

A: There are four things you need to do in conjunction with intermittent fasting to lose weight. If you feel like you're stuck and not losing weight, check these things off the list and make sure you're actually doing them.

1. **Use a Shorter Window:** One of the first things I do to escape a plateau is to decrease the length of my eating window. I'll add a few more 24-hour fast days to my week to increase my results. A 24-hour fast is easy for me to do. I can eat a meal at 1 p.m. and not eat again 1:30 p.m. the next day; that's a 24-hour fast.

2. **Wait for Stomach Growl** or wait for your stomach to get empty—Don't lose track of getting to true hunger. Your first meal of the day should never come before your stomach growl. There is a very small percentage of people who will be physically hungry but *won't* hear a growl.

3. **Eat When You're Hungry:** While you may not wait for a stomach growl to eat your second meal of the day, you should still be waiting until you're actually hungry to eat. We never eat unless we're hungry. Pay attention to your Hunger Scale. You should only eat your first meal at a 1 and your second meal at a 1-2.

4. **No Overeating:** This is the most important factor that you have to be honest with yourself about. You cannot overeat no matter what. If you're still eating too many calories, you're not going to lose weight no matter how much you fast.

You should only start looking at calories after you've confirmed that you're doing those four things. Take one week to evaluate what you're eating and what number of calories you should be consuming to lose the weight you want to lose. You might be surprised by how many calories are actually in the foods we eat. For example, there are 90 calories in just one tablespoon of peanut butter. That can add up if you're not careful.

Q: **What if I'm reaching the end of my six-hour window and my stomach isn't growling? Can I eat?**

A: Let's say you waited for your stomach to growl and you began your window at 12:30 p.m. Your window ends at 6:30 p.m., but maybe your stomach hasn't growled by the time your family is eating dinner at 5 p.m. Let's go back to that Hunger Scale. For the very first meal, you need to be at a 1 before you start your window. At your next meal (like the 5 p.m. family dinner), you can be a 2 and eat something really small. This way your stomach doesn't growl just after your window closes leaving you feeling tempted to eat.

Q: **What if I like to have coffee with cream in the morning?**

A: If you're the kind of person who lives for their coffee with cream every morning, you're going to have to make an adjustment for a little while. It is possible to have coffee with cream and no sugar every morning and still get results. If you decide to do that, just know that you may not get results as fast as someone else. This is because you're elevating your blood sugar when you drink that cup of coffee. I personally recommend you don't do it. However, if that is the one hang-up that's keeping you from starting this plan, then keep your coffee with cream. To be honest, when I was interviewing all of the thin eaters, almost all of them had coffee with a little creamer. Some had it black, but most had it with cream no sugar. Whatever you decide to do, it's best to wait and drink coffee 3-4 hours after you wake up or at least until you start getting hungry. Caffeine is an appetite suppressant, so when you drink it, it pushes you so that you can fast a little longer. On days when you're fasting but you feel like you just *have* to eat, that's when you drink the black coffee or unsweetened tea. Coffee can be very high in acid, so people who have a lot of digestive issues should try a low acid coffee, or just drink water if you have stomach acid issues.

Q: **Once I break the seal, I get out of control. Once I have one chip, I have to have**

20. Once I eat one French fry, I'm going to eat the whole thing! What if I don't know how to stop eating?

A: The reason you're out of control is that you've deprived yourself of the foods you want and you told yourself that these are "bad foods."

Yesterday, I went to Ocean Breeze Waterpark with my family. One of them got pizza, one got a hot dog, one got French fries, and they all got ice cream. I asked my husband for one bite of his pizza and it tasted disgusting. It was the worst thing! Then I had a French fry and I thought these are the worst fries ever! It was very easy to stop eating. The most I ate was three bites of ice cream. That goes back to the rule of decadent foods—just have a few bites.

The point is this: if I didn't have that stuff I would have been sitting there thinking, *I want that pizza! I want those fries!* Instead, I had one bite of all of them and thought *ehh*. I decided that the food was so disgusting that I wasn't going to eat. I wasn't starving-hungry, so it wasn't a problem. I've decided that I'm only going to fill my body with things I truly love. Why am I going to waste my calories on foods that are just *ehh*?

Q: **I have low blood sugar. Can I do intermittent fasting?**

A: I have had a major problem with low blood sugar, so I absolutely understand what it's like. I woke up this morning not feeling well, so around 8:30 a.m. I decided to take my blood sugar. It was 63. Anything under 70 is considered low, and when you're fasting your blood sugar should be between 80-100. I don't feel good when I'm in the 60-70 range. Now, remember, I'm not a doctor and this entire book is based on my personal experiences and what works for me. This is just my personal advice based on being someone who's had low blood sugar for a very long time. Consult your physician before making any change to your regular eating habits.

1. **Get a monitor.** First, you need to find out if you indeed have low blood sugar or if you're just constantly spiking and crashing because of a high-sugar diet. 1. Get yourself a continuous blood sugar monitor and test your blood sugar. If this is truly a problem for you, then you might want to eat smaller meals so that your stomach growls sooner and you can eat again.

2. **Move Around.** Typically, when you exercise your blood sugar drops, but I have found in my own experience that when my blood sugar is really low and I exercise and have some caffeine it actually goes back up. Do a little research and you'll find other people have a similar reactions.

3. **Drink unsweetened tea.** Like I said before, I woke up this morning with my

blood sugar at 63. I got up, walked around the house, and drank a glass of unsweetened tea. By 11 a.m., my blood sugar was 104, which is actually considered pre-diabetic. I went to Lucky Oyster later and had egg whites with spinach and onions as well as an egg and cheese biscuit with half of the biscuit removed. Twenty minutes after that meal, my blood sugar had only risen to 125. That's pretty good for it to only rise that much after eating a whole meal.

Unless your blood sugar is below 70, you shouldn't be eating when you're in your fasting window. Look, you're talking to the low blood sugar queen! If I can do it, so can you. You just have to check your blood sugar to see where it really is. Also, confirm you actually have a low blood sugar problem and that you aren't just addicted to sugar!

Q: **I want to try intermittent fasting, but I have low blood sugar. Can I go that long without eating?**

A: I had low blood sugar as well, so I absolutely understand what it's like. The crazy thing is intermittent fasting will actually help regulate your blood sugar. If you hang in there, you'll notice it gets better. If you begin Intermittent Fasting while having blood sugar issues, you'll need to do a good job of gradually weaning yourself off a long eating window. You may have to start with a 12-hour eating window, then step it down to 11, then 10, and so on. Intermittent fasting's effect on blood sugar is really fascinating.

Q: **I'm really concerned about doing intermittent fasting because I have low blood sugar. I'm afraid I'll pass out.**

A: First, you need to determine if you actually have low blood sugar. If it's just a fatigued feeling and not a doctor's diagnosis, it's probably what you're eating that makes you feel lethargic. If you eat a huge, carb-heavy lunch, it'll raise your blood sugar so high that when it comes back down, you "crash." Adjusting how you eat is important. More protein and fewer carbs are how I like to eat with intermittent fasting.

Q: **Aren't you going to eat so much more when you're in your eating window?**

A: In the beginning, I think you will. You'll have to remind yourself not to overeat. However, one of the benefits of fasting is that it gets you out of the habit of eating just because it's a certain time of day, and into the habit of eating only when you're hungry. It gets rid of the "I'm bored" snacking habit. That was a big deal for me. You have to be very careful not to eat out of boredom even if you are in your six-hour window.

Q: **What if I'm not seeing results?**

A: If you're not seeing results, the first question you need to ask yourself is, "What am I drinking?" Are you drinking Diet Coke, coffee with cream, flavored water with sugar in it? These are little things that can slow your weight loss. Believe it or not, they spike your insulin and that's something you don't want to do.

Keep in mind that losing weight takes time. I didn't lose anything for the first two weeks. That's why I don't recommend weighing yourself on a scale every day. Only weigh yourself once a week and at times when you're feeling really thin. Weighing yourself every day can discourage you.

Q: **Does this diet include a vegan option? If it doesn't, I'm not trying it. If it's not vegan, it can't be healthy!**

A: As long as you're following these other rules, you can be vegan if you want to be. Remember: *The Chantel Ray Way* is not a diet, so you can eat whatever you normally eat and that includes vegan. Genesis 9 makes it clear you can eat meat, but if you feel you need to eat vegan, then that is perfectly fine. The Bible tells us to be tolerant toward each other in what we eat (Romans 14:5).

Q: **How does the fasting window begin?**

A: If you're having trouble figuring out the beginning of your fasting window, remember that you are free to determine when you start and stop eating. The second you start eating, you're in your **eating window** and you are considered to be in the **fed state**. Your eating window is closed the minute you stop eating and the **fasting window** begins.

I talked to a girl this weekend who told me she wakes up in the morning starving but is not a dinner person. If you're like that, you may want to do a 9 a.m.-2 p.m. eating window. That's fine; that's your eating window. Your window is closed when you eat your very last bite.

Now, some people argue that when your fasting window begins, you're not really in a fasted state. For example, if you finished eating at 2 p.m., you're not immediately in a fasted state at 3 p.m. because your body is still fueling itself off the food you just ate. That's true, but it's not what we're talking about for the fasting window. We're dealing with **the time you're eating** vs. **the time you're fasting**. You get yourself to the fasted state by waiting until your stomach growls the next day. It's an accomplishment when your stomach growls because now you're really starting to burn fat.

Q: **What if I'm required to take food with my medication in the morning?**

A: Obviously, you'll have to break your fast in the morning, so you need to find something that will not cause your insulin to spike. Look for a high-fat food: something with cream or with a lot of butter. An egg is good as well. The yolk is very high-fat, low-carb. I would eat anything I could think of that was high-fat and low-carb, and I would eat as little of it in the morning as I could. Then I would wait for my stomach to growl before eating again. I definitely wouldn't try to have a whole meal. I wouldn't stress about it, but I would just make sure I had enough in my body so the medicine wouldn't mess up my stomach.

Q: **What about body odor?**

A: I had a friend tell me that once she started fasting, she was getting more intense body odor. She said her armpits and breath smelled more. That is just a matter of your body detoxing. Use a lot of mouthwash if your breath smells bad. Carry an extra deodorant with you in your purse for your armpits. It gets better, but right now your body is trying to get used to it. It may be kind of unpleasant, but you should really look at it as something that's good. It means you're doing a good thing for your body. Also, it causes an unexpected positive side effect: more showers! If you have a problem with eating impulsively, showers and baths are really good for you. They de-stresses you. If you're having an issue with body odor, use it as an opportunity to bathe instead of eating and increase your weight loss!

Q: **What if I'm not losing weight doing the eight-hour window?**

A: I've found that women have a hard time losing weight if they're only doing eight-hour eating windows. It's not enough fasting time and they're usually eating too much at each meal as well.

If you're working out, though, there may be another explanation. You may not be losing weight on the scale, but your body composition could be changing. Take me, for example, I am such a muscle builder. My mom used to smack me on the butt and call me the Rock of Gibraltar because I am just a solid piece of meat! There's a lot of muscle in my body. So, I have a jacket that I used to never be able to clasp both buttons, but now it fits just right! I'm not seeing the results I want when I get on the

ONE MEAL AND A TASTING

scale, but these other signs let me know my body is actually changing. Ultimately, you want to change your body composition more than you want to lose weight.

Q: Are artificial sweeteners harmful?

A: Here's the bottom line: you will not get the best results if you consume artificial sweeteners. The biggest area of struggle for most people is with drinking water. I have so many friends who say they hate water. They never drink it unless it's zero-calorie flavored water. However, I believe that when you do something for a few days, you just get used to it. For example, I used to always need some sort of Splenda in my tea because I thought unsweetened tea was disgusting. Now, I can drink my tea with no sweetener at all. It's something you'll get used to.

Q: Can I have artificial sweeteners during my eating window?

A: Once you're in your eating window, you can have them as much as you want. Do I like it? No! For me, artificial sweeteners are not good, and I'll never eat them. I don't like the way they taste, and if I'm going to eat something sweet, I want it to be real sugar. If you want to eat them, you're free to do so, but your results won't be as good.

If you do a web search on the effect of artificial sweeteners on blood sugar, you'll see competing results. I think it varies for every individual. Forget the studies and try it for yourself. If you're considering having artificial sweeteners in your diet, check your blood sugar before and after having them and see what happens.

Q: Are you getting enough calories when you eat one meal a day?

A: I'm sorry, but my aunt weighs 90 pounds, and she is never worried if she's getting enough calories! You're not going to ruin your metabolism by eating OMAD; that's a myth. You need to get this sort of thinking out of your mind. You are **not** overweight because you don't eat enough calories. Let's be honest with ourselves. That excuse is ludicrous, and it came from the diet industry.

Q: I'm not seeing my weight change on the scale. What's wrong?

A: I learned about something recently called the "whoosh effect." It explains why you don't always see a consistent change in your weight every day while you're burning fat. Because of the law of thermodynamics, burning more calories than you consume results in weight loss as your body gets the energy it needs from your fat reserves. This isn't a theory; it's actual physics. If you don't give your body food, it has to use the fat in your body. So, you may wonder why you can go a whole week and not lose weight when you know you were burning fat. That's where the "whoosh effect" comes in. It has to do with water retention. The idea is that your fat cells become filled with water as you're burning fat. Because of this, the scale doesn't change even though you did in fact burn fat. However, once your body finally drops that water (maybe 1-2 weeks later or more depending on the person) you lose a bunch of weight at once. That's called the "whoosh effect[1]." It's like the sound of your pounds being flushed down the toilet. Get it? It's not that you actually lost that many pounds overnight. It's that your weight loss finally "caught up" with your fat loss.

I didn't lose any weight at all during my first two weeks of doing this plan. In my third week, I lost six pounds, and in my fourth week, I lost four. *WHOOSH!* I lost all this weight! That's why I don't like getting on the scale every day. You're getting yourself worked up for no reason. Here's what I suggest as a better way to measure your weight loss: get a pair of pants that you don't ever wash or dry and try them on regularly to see how you're progressing. I even prefer this method to measuring your inches with measuring tape. When you use measuring tape, you have to be sure to measure the same exact spot and pull the tape just right every time or your reading won't be accurate.

Q: **I'm doing intermittent fasting and now I don't feel well. What am I doing wrong?**

A: Don't make the mistake of overdosing on the wrong foods just because you're allowed to eat whatever you want now. I've seen a lot of people who were eating really clean, but then went the complete opposite direction when they started intermittent fasting. Your body isn't going to feel well if you do that. This is why I focus on eating clean foods even if they're not "healthy." I know I have a high-fat diet. I don't worry about fat. I eat nuts that are high in fat, steak with butter, and all that stuff because the more fat I eat the better I feel. It's chemicals that I stay away from because I like to feel my best.

Q: **How do I know if I'm getting enough nutrients in my body?**

A: I take a lot of vitamins because I feel like the food we eat doesn't have as much as I need. Visit chantelrayway.com/vitamins.

Q: **What are your thoughts on having a cheat meal?**

---

1 Muir, Chris, "How Whooshes Impact Your Weight Loss" http://leanmuscleproject.com/how-whooshes-impact-your-weight-loss/
   Shellabarger, Brian. "The 'Whoosh' Effect" http://100down.org/the-whoosh-effect/
   "Of Whooshes and Squishy Fat" http://www.bodyrecomposition.com/fat-loss/of-whooshes-and-squishy-fat.html/

A: I don't call it a cheat meal because I eat what I want every day. On days when I'm not feeling great, I fill my body with super healthy foods to get my energy up.

Right now, I'm craving Baker's Crust's Gotta Have It burger. Since I want to keep it clean today, I'm going to take away the bun and wrap it in lettuce. When I need a lot of energy, I don't eat as many carbs. I'll eat red meat because my iron levels are lower than the average Joe. So, I'm going to have this burger wrapped in lettuce with some fries for potassium, and that will be my one meal for the day.

Q: What are your thoughts on alcohol and wine?

A: I went to a pool party last night and someone asked me if I wanted champagne. I told her no because I don't like to drink my calories. I have a ton of friends who do intermittent fasting and they really like to drink. The Bible says that Jesus drank wine, and I believe drinking is fine as long as you don't get drunk. There are also health benefits to drinking red wine. I'm a proponent of drinking wine if the Holy Spirit leads you to. I'm just not a drinker. I probably drink two to three times a year and I don't love it. I actually have this mental block against drinking because of all my years of dieting. It's this thought that if I don't drink my calories, I can have more to eat. I have plenty of friends who are very skinny and would much rather drink their calories than eat them. The main thing is that if you're drinking, you're doing it during your eating window. Go to www.chantelrayway.com/wine for more.

Q: But doesn't alcohol make you gain weight?

A: I have this group called the Thursday Funday group. I look at how much they eat and drink and they definitely increase their calories with alcohol. However, they are still as thin as they can be. Keep in mind most of those girls only eat one meal a day and a tasting. Most of them don't start eating before two or three in the afternoon, and they stay in that six or eight-hour window. Keep looking at the line between eating and overeating. If you are eating and drinking in your window, the alcohol should be fine.

Q: What are the benefits of red wine?

A: There are all kinds of studies explaining why you should drink red wine. They say it regulates your blood sugar. I don't really know because I don't drink it, but if Jesus drank it, I'm not going to look at you negatively for doing it. If you want to be literal, I suppose you could say you drink it to be more like Him. HAHA!

Q: How obsessive should I be on the eating window? If I started my window at 12:06 p.m., do I have to close it at exactly 6:06 p.m.?

A: Don't get obsessive! You don't have to pinpoint it to the exact minute. What you want is a consistent window to help you develop a routine, but this should never be stressful. Intermittent fasting is a tool that takes the stress out of your eating. If you start getting obsessive, then you're on the wrong track.

Q: If my eating window just opened, but I'm not truly hungry should I eat anyway?

A: No. If you're trying to lose weight, you definitely don't need to be forcing yourself to eat. Remember, we eat when we're truly hungry.

Q: I've read before that you should eat before you get hungry to avoid binging. Is that true?

A: If your car doesn't need gas, you don't put gas in it. If your bill isn't due, you don't pay money on it. I believe the same principle should apply to our bodies. I get the idea of trying to avoid binging, and, honestly, the first couple of weeks of intermittent fasting you'll probably overeat some. However, you will adjust.

Q: What are some tips to not overeat on your first meal of the day? Sometimes my work schedule is so busy that I can't take a break to eat. When I do finally begin my eating window, I'm starving.

A: Stay away from simple carbs and sugars on your first meal. Keep your digestion in mind and eat slowly. You're going to be full 20 minutes before you realize it, so don't rush through your meal just because you're hungry. Another great tip is to drink a glass of water an hour before you eat. This will take the edge off of the hunger so you can sit down and enjoy your meal without overeating. In fact, whenever you're feeling overwhelmed by hunger throughout the day, try drinking water. If it's been 45 minutes since your last drink, you could actually be dehydrated. Don't drink a ton of water while you're eating, though. You could dilute your stomach acids and hinder digestion.

Q: I'm so tired after eating my first meal of the day. Why am I so exhausted from fasting?

A: Are you eating too much? What are you eating? It's more likely that what you're eating is the source of the problem rather than the fasting. If you're eating whole, clean foods I have a hard time believing you're constantly tired, but perhaps you have an underlying health concern like anemia. Always stay in touch with your physician when you make any major changes to your eating patterns if you have a health condition.

Q: **I don't have enough energy to workout in my fasted state.**

A: There are a lot of possibilities. Are you getting enough of all of your proteins, carbs, and fats? Are you getting enough sleep? Maybe switch your workout time to be closer to your eating window so you can eat right after. Or, eat right before. I personally like to work out fasted, but everyone is different.

Q: **Are you allowed to lift heavy weights while fasting?**

A: I lift heavy weights every single morning in a fasted state. I've lifted heavier weights fasted than men in my gym! My trainer, Chris Sykes, tells me he does all of the same workouts he did before he started intermittent fasting and he hasn't lost any steam.

Made in the USA
Las Vegas, NV
30 August 2022